WORKING WITH BACKACHE

Marc T Rabideau

WORKING WITH BACKACHE

by Suzanne H. Rodgers, Ph.D.

Consultant in Ergonomics/Human Factors
Rochester, New York

Assistant Professor, Part-time, Physiology Department,
University of Rochester School of Medicine and Dentistry

Adjunct Associate Professor,
Industrial Engineering Department,
State University of New York at Buffalo

Illustrations by Leigh Ann Smith
Albany, New York

foreword by Stover H. Snook, Ph.D.
Project Director - Ergonomics
Liberty Mutual Insurance Company
Hopkinton, Massachusetts

Copyright © 1984 by Suzanne H. Rodgers, Ph.D.

Published July 1985
by
Perinton Press

All rights reserved. No part of this publication may be reproduced or transmitted in any form, by any means, electronic, magnetic, mechanical, photographic, or otherwise, including information storage and retrieval systems, without prior written permission from the publisher, except for brief quotations by a reviewer.

Library of Congress Catalog Card Number: 85-61915
ISBN 0-931-15701-3
Printed in the United States of America

FOREWORD

There is nothing new about backache. Bernardino Ramazzini, the founder of occupational medicine, was concerned about it back in 1690, and the ancient Egyptians suffered from it over 5000 years ago. The disorder appears to be as old as mankind itself - probably even older, since four-legged animals are also known to suffer from back problems. Over the centuries, medicine has not progressed as far in understanding and controlling low back pain as it has with other types of disorders. Consequently, as old as low back pain is, it remains a major source of impairment, disability and compensation in today's society.

Almost everyone suffers from low back pain at some time during their working career. Low back pain is generally defined as lumbosacral pain as well as buttock pain and leg pain; acute pain as well as chronic pain; and lumbago as well as lumbar insufficiency. It is generally recognized that low back pain of this nature is experienced by 80% of the population at some time during life.

Low back impairment represents a decrease or loss of ability to perform various musculoskeletal activities, and is very dependent upon the severity of low back pain. According to the National Center for Health Statistics, approximately 6 million Americans suffer from low back impairment at any one given time; a prevelance of almost 3 in every 100 people.

Low back disability is defined as time lost from the job, or assignment to restricted duty. Low back disability is very dependent upon the nature of the job. A person with low back impairment may not be able to perform a manual handling job, but may be able to perform a lighter job. According to studies from the Liberty Mutual Insurance Company, approximately 2% of American workers will suffer disabling low back pain every year.

Finally, low back compensation is reimbursement for lost wages, and is very dependent upon the nature of the compensation law. In the United States, compensation law varies from state to state. The same low back disability may be compensable in one state, but not in another. The important point is that low back pain may or may not involve low back impairment; low back impairment may or may not involve low back disability; and low back disability may or may not involve low back compensation.

There are many people who would like to believe that we can prevent low back pain. However, the objective evidence in the technical literature does not support that belief. Although we may not be able to prevent low back pain, we can reduce low back disability and compensation by training the patient, and redesigning the workplace and the job. Dr. Rodgers recognizes this fact by suggesting ways to work with low back pain. This is a very practical and humane approach to backache. It is practical because we can do it now without a major medical breakthrough. It is humane because many authorities now advocate activity and return to work as an important part of low back rehabilitation.

Some day we may be able to prevent low back pain, or at least substantially reduce it. Until then, our best approach is to learn how to work with backache - and this book will tell you how to do it.

    Stover H. Snook, Ph.D.
    Project Director - Ergonomics
    Liberty Mutual Insurance Company

PREFACE

Shortly after Dr. Rowe's important book, *Backache at Work*, was published in 1983, he presented a summary of his thoughts at an Occupational Safety Council meeting at the Rochester, N.Y. Chamber of Commerce. Although we had worked together at the Eastman Kodak Company for several years, I had not heard this encapsulated version of his thoughts on the low back pain problem in industry before, and I found his approach fascinating. It also fit with my own experience studying the occurrence and patterns of low back problems in the workplace associated with manual handling activities. In embracing Dr. Rowe's philosophy of the need to manage low back disability in industry, I began thinking about putting together a "how to" book relating ways to reduce job- and workplace design-related factors that might contribute to low back disability or time lost from work during low back pain episodes. *Working With Backache* is the result of those thoughts.

This book is written primarily for medical, safety, personnel, industrial hygiene, and engineering specialists who have to make decisions regarding occupational low back pain problems or who, through their design of the workplace and job, can influence factors that may contribute to low back pain symptoms. People with low back problems, including the author, have provided much of the pragmatic information contained herein, and future studies should give more attention to their approaches to limit the severity of repeat attacks.

Information from work physiology, manual handling, and biomechanics specialists has been simplified and generalized to make it fairly easy to use in evaluating existing workplaces or jobs. This simplification necessarily reduces accuracy in specific applications, so the reader is encouraged to learn the concepts but not be too strict in applying them to work situations. A universal rule in ergonomics is to try out an idea before you try to sell it, even if it looks good on paper. The guidelines included in this book are generally well-tested in the workplace, but inexpensive simulation of a new workplace or task design is the most effective way of "tweaking" it to assure that all factors have been considered. The most important concept in *Working With Backache* is that there are several ways to reduce low back disability and the symptoms of low back pain at work. The worker, management, and the designers of jobs can all contribute to an improved picture for people with low back pain. Through cooperative approaches to the problem, it should be possible to reduce time lost from work, improve productivity, and increase the comfort of people who are susceptible to repeated low back pain episodes.

      Suzanne H. Rodgers, Ph.D.
      Rochester, N.Y.
      February, 1985

ACKNOWLEDGMENTS

I am grateful to many people for their encouragement and helpful suggestions for ways to improve this book. Special thanks go to E. Carol Stein, M.D., Assistant Professor of Preventive, Family, and Rehabilitative Medicine and Director of Occupational Health Planning, University Health Service at the University of Rochester, for her careful review of the manuscript and suggestions for clarification of the text. Appreciation is also extended to David M. Kiser, Ph.D., Group Leader of the Ergonomics Group in Eastman Kodak's Health and Environment Laboratories, M. Laurens Rowe M.D., Consultant in Orthopaedic Surgery to Eastman Kodak Company (retired), Alice Rowe of Perinton Press, and to my father, John A. Rodgers for their critiques of the manuscript and helpful suggestions. The Foreword has been contributed by Stover Snook, Ph. D., Ergonomics Director of Liberty Mutual Insurance Company, to whom I am also grateful.

For their patience and enthusiasm for this project, Jim and Alice Rowe of Perinton Press deserve special thanks, as does the book's illustrator, Leigh Ann Smith of Albany, New York. I am also indebted to Shari Revell and Leslie Norton for typing the manuscript and doing other secretarial work.

For his encouragement and for educating me about low back problems prior to developing my own internal education system, I owe an additional big thank you to M. Laurens Rowe, M.D. My appreciation also goes to Robert H. Jones, M.D., Rehabilitation Consultant to Eastman Kodak Company, for teaching me about return-to-work problems and for many discussions about low back problems over the years. Thanks also to Harry L. Davis and Charles I. Miller, M.D., co-founders of the Human Factors Group at Eastman Kodak Company, who first introduced me to Ergonomics.

CONTENTS

Foreword v
Preface vii
Acknowledgements ix
Table of Contents xi
List of Figures xv
List of Tables xvi

Section I: Low Back Pain at Work

Chapter 1: The Management of Low Back Pain at Work 3
  A. Low Back Pain 4
    1. Incidence 4
    2. Diagnoses 6
    3. Natural History of Degenerative Disc Disease 6
  B. The Industrial Low Back Problem 9
    1. Relationship to Work 9
    2. Cost 10
    3. Approaches to Control Low Back Pain Disability ... 11
    4. Return to Work Problems 12

Section II: What the Worker Can Do

Chapter 2: Avoid Low Back Pain Aggravators 19
  A. Standing Workplaces - Postures 20
    1. Bending Over 21
    2. Hyperextension of the Back 22
    3. Extended Forward Reaches 23
    4. Crouching or Awkward Postures 28
    5. Constant Standing 26

B. Seated Workplaces - Postures 28
    1. Lack of Foot Support 28
    2. Twisting - Low Supply Cupboard 31
    3. Extended Forward Reaches 32
    4. Constant Sitting - Inadequate Support 33
  C. Manual Handling Tasks 34
    1. Heavy Lifting 35
    2. Twisting While Lifting or Pushing and Pulling 36
    3. Uneven Lifting or Carrying 39
    4. Handling an Over-Sized Load 41
    5. Sustained Heavy Handling or Awkward Postures ... 43

Chapter 3: Keep Muscles Fit 45
  A. Muscles That Support the Spine 45
  B. Muscle Strength and Fatigue 47
  C. Exercises to Keep These Muscles Fit 48
    1. Bent Knees Abdominal Curl 49
    2. Leg Pull 50
    3. Cross-Over Stretch 50
    4. Whole Body Stretch 50
    5. Side Slides 50

Chapter 4: Lift Safely 53
  A. Safe Lifting and Low Back Pain 53
  B. General Lifting Guidelines.......................... 54
    1. Do Not Twist While Lifting 54
    2. Plan the Lift 56
    3. Determine the Best Lifting Technique 56
    4. Take a Secure Grip on the Object Being Handled .. 59
    5. Pull the Load in Close to Your Body 59
    6. Alternate Lifting Tasks With Lighter Work 60
  C. Other Manual Handling Techniques.................. 60
    1. Two-Person Lifting 61
    2. Sliding and Pushing 61

Section III: How the Workplace Can Be Improved

Chapter 5: Work Location - Heights and Distances 65
  A. Location and Body Mechanics 66
  B. Working Heights and Reaches 69
  C. Orientation of the Workplace 75

Chapter 6: Seating 79
  A. Types of Workplaces - Standing, Sitting,
     and Sit/Stand 79
  B. Chair Design 81
    1. Chair Seat Height Adjustability 81
    2. Chair Seat Width 83
    3. Chair Seat Length or Depth 83
    4. Chair Seat Slope 84
    5. Chair Backrest 84
    6. Other Characteristics - Swivel, Support, Covering .. 87
  C. Footrests and Armrests 88

Chapter 7: Design of Manual Handling Tasks 91
  A. Association of Manual Handling and Low Back Pain .. 91
  B. Handling Location 92
  C. Lifting Guidelines to Reduce
     Low Back Pain Aggravation 98
    1. Occasional Lifts - The NIOSH
      Manual Lifting Guidelines 98
    2. Frequent Lifts 101
  D. Force Exertion Guidelines 104

Chapter 8: Special Workplace Aids for People with Low
       Back Pain 109
  A. Workplace Postures 109
    1. To Reduce Forward Bending and
      Extended Reaches 109
    2. To Reduce Hyperextension of the Back 111
    3. To Reduce Twisting 112
    4. To Provide Postural Relief in Constant
      Sitting or Standing Jobs 113
  B. Manual Materials Handling Aids 114
    1. Improving Body Postures
      During Handling Tasks 115
    2. Reducing the Amount of Work in
      Handling Objects 118

Section IV: How the Job Can Be Improved

Chapter 9: The Size and Design of
       Objects to Be Handled 123

   A. Dimensions of the Load 124
   B. Configuration of the Load 127
   C. Design of Handholds 129

Chapter 10: Providing Adequate Recovery Time 131
   A. Muscle Fatigue and Spinal Stability 131
   B. Postural Relief 133
   C. Manual Handling Tasks and Recovery Needs 135
   D. Examples of Recovery Time Calculations 137
      1. Static Muscle Loading 137
      2. Dynamic Work - Repetitive Manual Lifting 138

Chapter 11: Work Patterns and Job Design 143
   A. Work and Recovery Patterns in Self-Paced Work 143
   B. Paced Work and Work Patterns 145
   C. Job Design Guidelines 146

Section V: Summary and Addenda

Chapter 12: Summary 149
   A. New Design 150
   B. Existing Workplaces 151

Appendix A: Surveying the Workplace 155
   1. Checklist to Identify Potential Low Back Pain
      Aggravators in the Workplace 155
   2. Other Factors to Evaluate in the Workplace 158

Appendix B: Selecting a Chair 161
   1. Chair Characteristics as Selection Criteria 161
   2. The Process of Chair Selection 161

References 169

Index 175

Contents

LIST OF FIGURES

Figure I-1: Low Back Pain in Industry 5
Figure I-2: The Natural History of
Degenerative Disc Disease 8
Figure II-1: Bending 21
Figure II-2: Hyperextension of the Back 22
Figure II-3: Extended Forward Reaches 24
Figure II-4: Awkward Postures 25
Figure II-5: Lack of Foot Support 28
Figure II-6: Twisting in a Seated Workplace 30
Figure II-7: Twisting While Lifting 37
Figure II-8: Uneven Load Carriage 40
Figure II-9: Over-Sized Load Handling 42
Figure II-10: Muscles Supporting the Lower Spine 46
Figure II-11: Static Work Intensity
and Duration Relationship 48
Figure II-12: Bent-Knees Abdominal Curl 49
Figure II-13: Four Back Strengthening Exercises 51
Figure II-14: Guidelines for Lifting 55
Figure II-15: Bent Knees and Derrick Lifting Styles 57
Figure II-16: Position of the Feet in Low Lifting 58
Figure III-1: Load Location and
Forward Bending Moment 68
Figure III-2: Standing Anthropometric Measurements 70
Figure III-3: Seated Anthropometric Measurements 71
Figure III-4: Standing Forward Reach Capability 73
Figure III-5: Seated Forward Reach Capability 74
Figure III-6: Workplace Orientation in a Packing Task 76
Figure III-7: Recommended Seating Design 82
Figure III-8: Work Location and Backrest Utilization
in a Seated Workplace 85
Figure III-9: Molded and Tubular Chair Design 86
Figure III-10: Good and Poor Handling Locations 93
Figure III-11: Relative Static Pull Strength and Location -
Males 95
Figure III-12: Relative Static Pull Strength and Location -
Females 96
Figure III-13: Lifting Height Design 97
Figure III-14: NIOSH Manual Lifting Guidelines 99
Figure III-15: Aerobic Work Intensity and
Duration Relationship 103

Figure III-16: Guidelines for Repetitive Lifting 105
Figure III-17: Examples of Force Applications 107
Figure III-18: Reach Extenders 110
Figure III-19: Height Adjustments for the Worker 111
Figure III-20: Use of Roller Bearing and Roller Conveyor
               Sections to Reduce Handling Effort 112
Figure III-21: Back Support Aids for Seated Work 114
Figure III-22: Postural Relief Aids at a
               Standing Workplace 115
Figure III-23: A Special Aid for Large-Size
               Sheet Handling 116
Figure III-24: Aids to Support an Object's Weight During
               Transfer Tasks 117
Figure III-25: A Load Levelling Aid for Manual
               Handling Tasks 118

Figure IV-1: Effect of Object Length on Elbow Position 124
Figure IV-2: Object Width and Back and
             Shoulder Posture 125
Figure IV-3: Object Depth and One-Handed
             Carrying Postures 126
Figure IV-4: Load Configurations 128
Figure IV-5: Recovery Times as a Function of Work
             Intensity and Duration 134
Figure IV-6: Lifting Patterns for People With and
             Without Low Back Pain 144

Figure B-1: Selecting a Chair 164

LIST OF TABLES

Table I-1: Return to Work Considerations 13
Table III-1: Maximum Force
             Application Recommendations 106
Table IV-1: Heart Rate Elevations in Several
            Occupational Tasks 139
Table B-1: Recommended Chair and
           Accessory Characteristics 162
Table B-2: Chair Selection By Job Category 165

Section I: Low Back Pain at Work

Chapter 1: The Management of Low Back Pain at Work

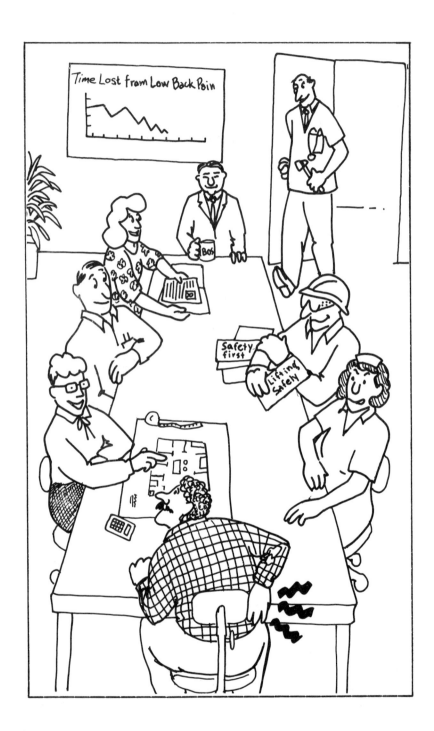

Section I:
Low Back Pain at Work

CHAPTER 1:
THE MANAGEMENT OF LOW BACK PAIN AT WORK

Most industrial safety or loss control managers will acknowledge that low back pain is the single most important factor in Workers' Compensation costs. Despite long-standing attempts to reduce the incidence of low back problems, first through lifting programs taught by safety personnel, and more recently through pre-placement strength testing, the low back problem has not significantly abated. Experts in the field are rethinking the earlier premise that low back pain can be "prevented" by teaching people how to lift properly and by using only the strongest people on heavy lifting jobs.

In *Backache at Work,* Dr. M.L. Rowe suggests that a more appropriate approach to low back pain in industry is to accept the fact that 56% or more of the workers will report symptoms at some time during their working careers. Hence, the institution of programs to manage the disability associated with degenerative disc disease, the most common cause of low back pain, should do more to control low back compensation costs than either lifting training or selection testing have done. In this chapter low back pain is discussed, especially in relation to the natural history of degenerative disc disease. It is viewed in the context of how low back pain affects industry and what is being done to control it. Finally, an introduction to the rest of the book reviews ways in which the worker, workplace designers, and management can help manage low back pain disability so the worker can continue to work, even with back pain.

A. LOW BACK PAIN

The studies by Dr. M.L. Rowe at Eastman Kodak Company have been reported in several papers and in *Backache at Work*. These longitudinal studies are unique in that one person was able to follow over 1500 men during a 20-year period and observe the pattern of low back pain events during that time. From data gathered in Rowe's 8 studies, an understanding of the incidence, diagnoses, and the natural history of degenerative disc disease has been developed.

1. Incidence

Statistics on the incidence of low back pain in industry vary widely. The number of people who actually lose time from work because of back pain will be less than the number of workers reporting back pain to a company medical department over a specific period; both will be considerably less than the number who report it on a questionnaire in which people are asked if they have ever had back pain.

Three of the studies reported by Rowe (1983) can be used to evaluate the incidence of low back pain in an industry with both light and heavy work (Figure I-1). In a review of all first visits to the Medical Department in one year, 5.5% of the plant population was seen for low back pain. This represented 5.8% of the male and 4.4% of the female workers in all jobs. Of these men and women, 68% could not identify a particular event that produced the low back pain and 16% identified an event outside of the workplace. The remaining 16% ascribed the back pain to some event at work. Only about 15% of these low back Workers' Compensation cases resulted in extended absence or in disability due to low back pain.

In a review of 237 male retirees (ages 62-65) with a long work history at the company, Rowe found that 56% had had low back pain severe enough to report to the Medical Department during their working years, and half of them had lost time from work because of it. In a ten-year study of male workers in one

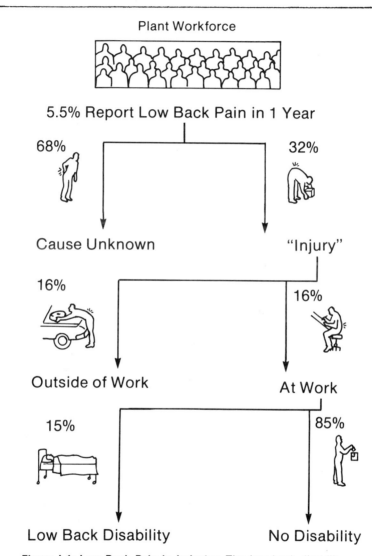

Figure I-1: Low Back Pain in Industry. The low back disability picture shown is based on over 1600 first reports to a Medical Department during one year. The breakdown by percent of reports that were attributed to an injury either on the job or at home is shown. Workers' Compensation reports indicate that 15% of the people reporting work-related "injuries" to the back may develop some disability.

production division, 47% of the men in heavy jobs reported to the Medical Department with low back pain and 22% lost time from work. Thirty-five percent of the men in lighter jobs also reported low back pain and 14% lost time.

Based on these studies, it appears that at least half of the employees in a plant will experience low back pain sometime in their working lives, and perhaps half of them will lose work time because of it.

2. Diagnoses

Low back pain is a symptom that may result from many causes. These include functional or developmental abnormalities, degeneration of discs or spinal facet joints, injuries, and tumors of the spine. It may be a referred pain from abdominal or pelvic organs, such as the gastrointestinal tract and the genito-urinary organs. In his study of over 1500 male employees over a 20-year period, Rowe (1983) found the following clustering of diagnoses to account for low back pain symptoms:

Disc degeneration and sequellae - 68%
(including abnormal motion between the vertebrae, facet joint subluxation, reactive bony productive changes, disc protrusion, and degenerative spondylolisthesis).

Inflammation - 20%
(including arthritis, prostatitis, and anklylosing spondylitis).

Miscellaneious Causes - 8%
(including developmental spondylolisthesis and situational causes where no disease can be detected).

True Injury - 4%

A detailed analysis of these diagnoses and their presentation in a patient with low back pain can be found in "Backache at Work."

3. Natural History of Degenerative Disc Disease

Because 68% of low back pain diagnoses in the Rowe study

The Management of Low Back Pain at Work 7

are attributed to degenerative disc disease, it is useful to describe the natural history of this disease with the hope that activities that exacerbate low back pain symptoms can be avoided.

In degenerative disc disease microscopic tears and ravelings occur in the disc casing fibers, usually in the posterior third of either the L4 or L5 disc (lumbar spine). Because the disc lacks a blood supply, it cannot repair itself. These tears accumulate and may eventually result in sufficient weakening of the disc casing to allow fluid leakage from the pressurized gel that makes up the disc. This "flattens" the disc somewhat and destablilizes the coupling between the vertebrae on either side of the disc, making it less rigid, or "sloppy." The vertebrae then can slide out of alignment and may pinch the dorsal nerve root that passes between the vertebrae (see Rowe, 1983 for illustrations and discussion of the pathomechanics of degenerative disc disease). Movements of the trunk that encourage movement in these less rigid vertebral couplings further destabilize them; so for example, twisting or leaning forward to pick up a load can further damage the disc casing. Actual disc herniation probably occurs in less than 5% of the cases of disc involvement. However, it may require surgical intervention to relieve pressure on the nerve root.

The natural history of five decades of degenerative disc disease symptoms is shown in Figure I-2. The initial attacks may occur when a person is in his or her 20's. These are usually mild and diffuse but may represent early increments of damage to the disc casing fibers. The attacks tend to be short and the symptoms usually totally disappear between them. In the 30's and 40's, there are more frequent attacks. These tend to be more severe, resulting in more lost time and some disability. The pain becomes more localized and lateralizes to one side. This is indicative of pressure on a nerve root with abnormal sensations, numbness, and pain usually following the distribution of the sciatic nerve. Residual pain is often present between acute attacks. In the 50's, the symptoms tend to settle into more of an arthritic pattern, one exacerbated by temperature and humidity changes and relieved by activity. By the time a person reaches his or her 60's, connective tissue has stabilized the vertebrae around the damaged disc and more activity may be tolerable than had been during the previous three decades.

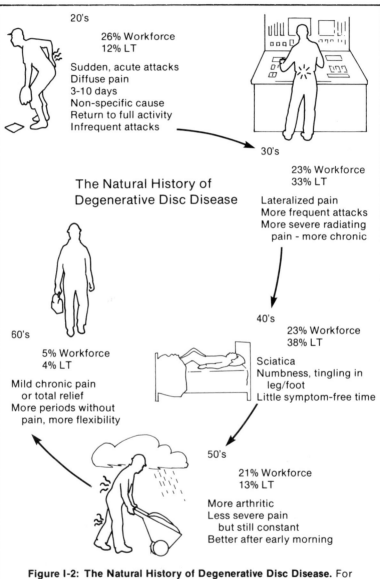

Figure I-2: The Natural History of Degenerative Disc Disease. For each decade between the 20's and the 60's, the symptoms of low back problems are listed. The % of the workforce in those decades and the % of lost time (% LT) from work due to low back pain is also shown. The exposure risk data are taken from the studies of Dr. Rowe (1983) over a 20-year period.

B. THE INDUSTRIAL LOW BACK PROBLEM

From the previous section, it is clear that many employees can be expected to experience low back pain during their working years. One may not be able to prevent the occurrence of degenerative disc disease, but it may be possible to lessen its clinical severity and to reduce the amount of disability experienced by 15% of the workers who account for 80% of the total compensation costs to industry (Rowe, 1983). This section addresses the relationship between low back pain incidence and job heaviness, the cost of low back pain to industry, methods used in attempting to control the problem, and some of the problems associated with returning a person with degenerative disc disease to work.

1. Relationship to Work

Rowe's analysis of one production divisions' medical records (1983) suggests that people in heavy effort jobs report more low back pain than do those in light effort jobs. Heavy effort in this example is lifting objects weighing about 40-50 lb (18-22 kg) on a fairly repetitive basis, usually 6 times per minute for 10 minutes continuously, repeated about 6 times per shift. Other occasional lifting of supplies or pushing and pulling of handcarts may also occur between the more frequent lifting activities. Forty seven percent of the male workers on the heavy effort jobs reported to the Medical Department in a 10-year period with low back pain symptoms, and 22% of them lost some time. This compared to 35% of the people in light effort jobs, 14% of whom lost time from work for low back pain. This difference in low back pain incidence between the workers in light and in heavy effort jobs is less than might have been anticipated. Rowe (1983) attributed the higher reporting and lost time for people in heavier jobs to a "need to report" back pain. This theory was supported by the observation that departments reporting more back pain also report more upper respiratory infections, gastrointestinal disturbances and all other diagnoses than are reported by the general plant population.

In a study of 100 consecutive Workers' Compensation cases for low back pain, Rowe (1983) found that 76% of the people were doing their accustomed work when the back pain occurred. Twelve percent of the cases could be directly related to an injury; 8% were associated with an unguarded move, and only 4% were associated with unaccustomed work. This contradicts the argument that low back injuries at work are often sustained when a person is doing heavy work to which he or she is not accustomed. Although these conditions doubtless contribute to the industrial low back pain problem, they are probably not the decisive factor in its etiology. Yet, it is the heavy job to which most of the efforts to control back problems have heretofore been directed, through teaching people how to lift, setting weight lifting limits, and using strength testing to select people with enough strength to match the measured job demands.

It appears that people who work in heavy effort jobs, in workplaces where postural demands are heavy, or where sustained awkward motions are required, are less able to continue that work during an episode of low back pain. Conversely, people in more sedentary jobs who can control their postures and workloads are less likely to need relief from job demands when they have low back pain. One way to reduce lost time associated with back pain is, therefore, to provide workplace aids or designs that lessen the likelihood of aggravating the vulnerable back and that enable people to work with some backache. These "aggravators" are discussed in Chapter 2.

2. Cost

The cost of low back pain to industry is often expressed in terms of Workers' Compensation payments. This represents only a fraction of the actual cost. Low back pain is variously described as costing the industrial sector 1 to 7 billion dollars a year (White, 1983), even though the compensation costs are considerably lower than that. About one-third of the Workers' Compensation costs are related to low back pain, however, and, of those, about 15% of the people account for 80% of the cost (Rowe, 1983). These low back disability cases are often people in their 30's and 40's who are unable to return to their jobs. Because of their youth, they may be on disability for up to 35 years, representing a large and continuing cost to industry. It is obviously to the advantage of the individual with low back disability as well as to industry to attempt to reduce the incidence and severity of the disability and to return the worker to a productive role as soon as possible.

Like many other "costs" in industry, the actual cost of low back pain is more than the compensation and disability dollars and time lost from work. Personal productivity may be reduced for a worker who is experiencing an episode of low back pain or for a person who has the residual backache seen between episodes in more advanced degenerative disc disease. This can occur if the pain is distracting, requiring a worker to change posture frequently, stretch, and take recovery breaks from heavy lifting tasks or sustained postures. Additional costs include training others to fill in for a person disabled with back pain, and those of company medical, supervisory, and personnel time spent trying to determine when the person can return to work and what work restrictions will be needed.

Since about 75% of the people with low back pain have repetitive episodes (Rowe, 1983), the opportunities for costs to accrue are vast. The control of these costs by managing the degree of disability of a person with backache is the focus of this book.

3. Approaches to Control Low Back Pain Disability

Over the past 50 years there have been a number of approaches made to control the industrial low back pain problem. These can be grouped into four categories: the selection of workers for the heavier jobs; education on safe handling of materials; the setting of weight limits along with workplace and job design to accommodate workers with less strength; and the development of exercise and behavior modification programs ("Back Schools") to help the worker with low back pain learn to cope with any disability. Workplace modification may also be part of the last program.

Recognizing that low back pain disability often cannot be linked to a particular action, some medical departments report back incidents in two ways: those where an "injury" is identified; and those where there appears to be a "physical failure," not attributable to any workplace condition or job demand. An example of physical failure of the back is when a person bends over to tie a shoe and cannot straighten up again. From Rowe's studies (1983), it is possible that about 75% of the compensable back problems can be classified as physical failures.

The above strategies to control low back disability are discussed briefly in later sections of this book. Over the past ten years the emphasis has been slowly evolving from one of prevention of low back pain incidents through training, selection, and enforcement of weight limits, to that of active intervention in the low back pain case in order to prevent long-term disability; this is the fourth strategy mentioned above.

4. Return to Work Problems

The factors that need to be addressed in order to reduce low back-related lost time in industry are grouped in Table I-1 according to who can do something about them: the worker with low back pain, supervision in the department of concern and other management personnel, and the job and workplace designers. Clearly, individuals with more severe degenerative disc disease may find it more difficult to return to work.

For the worker, the following factors may influence his or her return to work after a prolonged absence associated with low back pain:

- degree of disability, including postural muscle weakness resulting from the enforced inactivity during the attack

- financial incentives or disincentives

- alternative skills available for a job change

- job satisfaction before the incident

A worker who can make more money on disability than at work, who has limited alternative job skills and needs to be restricted from much of the work he or she has been doing, or who is not particularly content with his or her job represents a poor risk for prompt return to work.

Table I-1: Return to Work Considerations

Person(s) With Control	Factors
Worker	Degree of Disability Other Medical Problems Motivation/Illness Behavior Alternative Skills
Workplace and Job Designers	Postures Required Manual Handling Required Durations of Heavy Tasks or Awkward Postures Job Pattern Control by Worker Accommodations Available
Administrators/ Supervisors	Worker's Previous Job Performance Flexibility in Job Methods Availability of Other Jobs Production Pressures Training Programs Benefits Structure

Table I-1: Return to Work Considerations. Some factors are listed that may influence the ease with which a person with degenerative disc disease can return to work after an attack of low back pain. These are factors that determine the size of the disability problem from low back problems in industry. The workplace and job factors are discussed in more detail in this book.

The worker's supervision or other company management can affect the worker's ability to return to work. For example, by:

- making available other jobs within the worker's skill-level and not requiring extensive retraining or significant salary reductions

- showing flexibility in looking for job accommodations to help the worker back to his or her old job

- providing auxiliary help for occasional tasks that may be difficult for the worker with back pain to perform alone

- providing training to help develop the worker's alternative job skills

- providing a rehabilitation exercise program if absence from work is longer than 3 weeks.

A supervisor who must generate a certain amount of product per shift, day, or week may resist returning someone to work who can do only part of the job, especially if there are many people available in the outside labor force who can do the full job with a minimum of training. Returning a person with significant degenerative disc disease to a physically demanding job that takes only a few months to learn, such as loading tractor trailers with shipping cases or handling supplies in a stockroom, can be especially difficult. The job demands are more likely to aggravate the worker's symptoms, and restrictions from heavy lifting will most likely be requested by the worker's personal physician. Both the availability of alternative jobs and the ways in which the task can be altered to accommodate the worker with low back disability may also be limited.

The worker who has been an excellent and valued team member before the back problem occurred will be more likely to be accommodated than one with a mediocre work record. If the low back pain victim is considered to have "caused" his or her own problem by doing something careless ("didn't lift safely"), supervision may deny that worker the opportunity to return to work until the whole job can be performed. And although it is

The Management of Low Back Pain at Work

probably incorrect to say that the back problem was "caused" by improper lifting, this is often said in heavy jobs.

The job and workplace designers can influence the cost of low back disability by modifying the following factors:

- the postural demands of work - whether the worker has to maintain awkward or fatiguing postures in order to operate the machine, asemble the parts, or do the tasks required on the job

- the seating available - its design and appropriateness for a person with low back problems (backrest, foot support, etc.)

- provision of recovery periods after heavy work or sustained awkward postures

- inclusion of workplace accommodations such as support stools, footrails, or adjustable height tables to permit the person with low back disability to get postural relief during sustained work

- provision of handling aids to reduce the lifting and carrying demands of jobs

- reduction of unnecessary manual handling tasks through a systems approach to materials handling that uses conveyors and automated equipment, when appropriate.

All such design factors can make it easier for the person with some low back disability to return to work. The reduction of job effort demands should permit this worker to do much of the job when the back pain is not severe. Factors that aggravate the low back pain symptoms are also reduced; hence there is a lessened need to report them. Most of this job design work is best done during initial facility layouts and job specifications. Designing jobs and workplaces to accommodate a majority of the potential work force will make them more suitable for people with low back pain as well. If the job and workplace are already designed, accommodations or aids may often be added at low cost, with solutions limited only by the creativity of the designer and workers in the area.

In the remainder of this book, the roles of the worker, supervision, and designers are discussed in more detail. Specific recommendations are given for workplace accommodations and job design that will help the person with low back pain remain an active member of the workforce for most of his or her career.

Section II: What the Worker Can Do

Chapter 2: Avoid Low Back Pain Aggravators

Chapter 3: Keep Muscles Fit

Chapter 4: Lift Safely

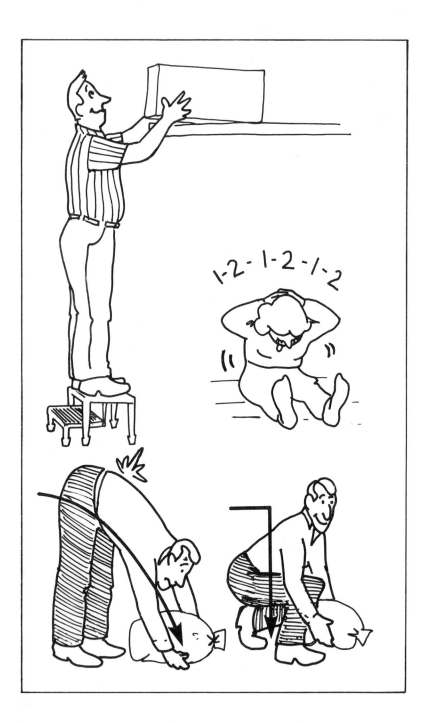

Section II:
What the Worker Can Do

There are actions that the worker can take to avoid aggravating underlying degenerative disc disease. Most people with chronic back problems know intuitively what these are, although they may not be able to formally define them. These actions must be avoided both at work and at home, and examples of each are included in Chapter 2. Exercises to keep the trunk and limb muscles fit are included in Chapter 3 as another means the worker can take to reduce the frequency and severity of low back pain. Chapter 4 includes information about techniques for manual handling; these reduce the stress on the L4 and L5 discs and make overexertion incidents less likely to occur.

CHAPTER 2: AVOID LOW BACK PAIN AGGRAVATORS

The characteristic symptoms of degenerative disc disease have been described briefly in Chapter 1 and thoroughly in *Backache at Work* by Dr. M.L. Rowe (1983). The microscopic tears and ravelings in the L4 and L5 disc casing that can lead to fluid leakage and the "sloppy" vertebral linkages in this area may be increased by postures and manual handling activities that put high compressive or shear forces on the disc, especially on the posterior one-third of the disc near the nerve roots. Once a person is in the more advanced stages of degenerative disc disease, certain motions or actions may trap the nerve root between two vertebrae, or may stretch or tear the capsule or the ligaments of the facet joints between the vertebrae. High forces on the disc may cause it to rupture and press on the nerve root. All of these can result in severe pain. Some of these motions are described and illustrated in this chapter. In addition to increasing the compressive and shear forces on the disc and increasing the instability of the vertebrae in the L4 or L5 area, these motions increase muscle fatigue, thereby reducing a person's ability to "protect" the back. These factors are discussed under standing and seated workplace postures and manual handling tasks. They represent actions that the worker with chronic backache should avoid. It is no doubt safer for the person without backache as well to avoid continued exposure to these activities. Although the worker has some control over the actions he or she takes when away from work, the same options may not be available in the workplace. Sections III and IV show how the workplace and job can be designed or altered to reduce the tasks that can aggravate low back pain symptoms.

A. Standing Workplaces - Postures

Although a great deal of emphasis has been placed on the role of manual materials handling activities in the etiology or aggravation of low back pain, postural factors are probably at least equally important. In a standing workplace, there are many factors to consider when looking for actions that may increase back pain symptoms. These include:

- bending over, unsupported by the arms, as in work at a drafting board

- hyperextending the back, as in high reaches

- extended forward reaches

- crouching or other awkward postures, such as leaning to one side

- constant standing

They are discussed in the context of how they influence the lumbar spine in a person with degenerative disc disease.

Avoid Low Back Pain Aggravators 21

1. Bending Over

Figure II-1 illustrates the posture of a person doing food preparation in a kitchen. Because the work involves downward forces, the counter is 36 inches (90 cm) high, although the visual demands of the work would be better satisfied with a 43-inch (110 cm) high work surface. The worker bends over to exert the necessary force and to have good visual control of the task. This statically loads the back and hip muscles. At the same time, the weight of the upper body is now acting as a load on the spine because it is no longer aligned over the feet. The back muscles have a very short lever arm (2 inches or 5 cm) and are quite heavily loaded in the bending posture (see Chapter 5 for further discussion of biomechanical stresses on the back). This static loading can fatigue the muscles that stabilize the back in response to forward flexion of the trunk. The longer this posture must be sustained, the more fatigue will accumulate. There is then more opportunity for the back to be "unprotected" by these fatigues muscles when a twisting motion, uneven weight distribution, or unexpected motion occurs.

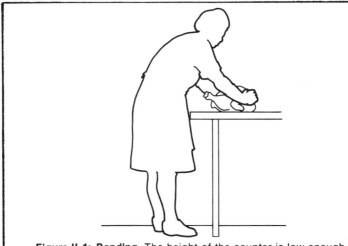

Figure II-1: Bending. The height of the counter is low enough to require the kitchen attendant to bend over from the hips while preparing the turkey. This bending loads the hip extensors and the erector spinae muscles that extend the trunk and will fatigue them if it is sustained for a minute or more.

Besides work done on a low counter, bending over may be required when a person has to work in an area with inadequate head clearance. This situation may occur fairly frequently for maintenance workers, caisson workers, coal miners, and people who load and unload shelving units that are less than 6 feet (2 meters) high. These requirements for bending are more difficult for the worker to avoid than a too-low counter surface where, for example, thickness may be added to the surface by using sheets of plywood or other materials to build up the height for better visual access. For too-low head clearance, the worker can only avoid sustained work in the bent-over posture by taking small sitting or lying down breaks to relieve the static back muscle stress or by working from a kneeling posture, where appropriate.

2. Hyperextension of the Back

An example of an activity that produces hyperextension of the back is illustrated in Figure II-2. Hyperextension involves moving the trunk past its normal erect position so that the upper body is oriented behind its normal resting point. As the spine extends backwards, the pelvis moves forward, and there is a

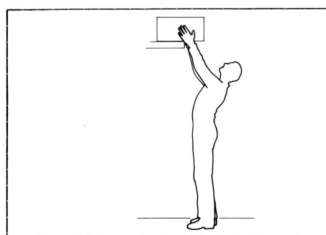

Figure II-2: Hyperextension of the Back. The need to reach or handle materials from locations over shoulder height usually results in arching, or hyperextension, of the back. This increases the load on the posterior third of the lumbar discs and may result in back pain symptoms in susceptible people.

concentration of compressive force on the posterior one-third of the L4 or L5 discs. This increased pressure can aggravate an already damaged disc and may result in a pinched nerve root if the lower vertebra's articular process slides forward and partially closes off the nerve root's exit port. Even for persons with no history of degenerative disc disease, repeated hyperextension of the back, especially during manual handling tasks, is not recommended since it may increase the rate of microscopic tear and raveling damage to the normal disc casing.

Activities that cause hyperextension are primarily those involving tasks above shoulder height, i.e., about 52 inches (132 cm) above the floor. The tasks include reading dials or displays located above standing eye height, about 60 inches (150 cm) above the floor. The person who is handling cases or products with the back hyperextended is putting additional stress on the lumbar discs. A person who sometimes works lying on the stomach in order to access the task, such as the case of a low-seam coal miner, a maintenance worker fixing a machine, or an automobile mechanic, may also hyperextend the back when his or her head is raised. Finally, many extended reaches (discussed below) are accompanied by back hyperextension.

The worker can control the amount of hyperextension in many overhead tasks by using a step stool or platforms or by avoiding the placement of materials over shoulder height where there is a choice. Where the hyperextension is associated with work on the stomach, frequent short recovery breaks are recommended to rest the back and abdominal muscles between exertions.

3. Extended Forward Reaches

Reaches that exceed the length of a person's arm and require bending or stretching forward to accomplish a task can aggravate low back pain in several ways: forward stretches can result in hyperextension of the back to counteract the tendency to fall forward; unequal loading of the spine can occur if only one hand and arm are used in the activity; bending forward puts a mechanical stress on the lower back; and the handling of any weight or exertion of any force at full arm's extension can put high compressive and/or shear force on the lumbar intervertebral discs because of the posture and long force arm (see Figure II-3).

Extended reaches with both arms or unequal stretching of one arm forward in a task can occur in many occupational tasks. Large-size objects may create extended reaches, as will be discussed in Chapters 7 and 9. Activation of valves, reaches across work stations to get supplies or to pull materials off of a conveyor, and reaches into the far corner of a large shipping case represent activities where extended reaches are often required. At home, reaching to the upper shelf in a cupboard, trying to remove the tire and jack from the trunk of a large car, and tree trimming often involve extended and unbalanced reaches that can aggravate low back symptoms.

A worker can avoid some of these reaches by using handle extenders on inaccessible valves (illustrated in Chapter 8), and using aids to activate distant controls. To move an object closer one can sometimes slide it forward using a "crook" or "hook." Some reaches can be reduced by tilting the case or product container upward by 15 to 30 degrees, the far side being uphill of

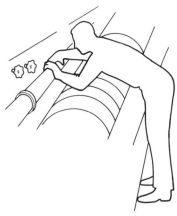

Figure II-3: Extended Forward Reach. Reaches that are more than 20 inches in front of the body or are below standing waist level will require the worker to bend at the waist and put additional pressure on the lower back. If part of the workplace or equipment makes it difficult to bend the knees, the stress on the lumbar discs is greater.

the near side at the workplace. Because the greatest arm reach is at shoulder level, postural adjustments such as bending the knees or using a step stool to keep the reach at shoulder level comprise another strategy to reduce aggravation of low back symptoms during extended reaches.

4. Crouching or Awkward Postures

Some occupational tasks require crouching, stooping, or leaning over, all of which put a load on the low back and its lumbar discs. Figure II-4 illustrates a welder in a crouching position; this can be a fairly acceptable posture for short periods of time. Sustained work in this posture, with some shifting of the body weight to maintain stability, can put strong shear and compressive forces on the lumbar discs as the back muscles stabilize the posture during forward bending of the trunk. When a person stands up after an extended period in a crouched posture, the muscles of the back may not support the spine as well (due to fatigue), increasing the likelihood of a pinched nerve root.

Postures where one hip is higher than the other, or where a load is not borne evenly across the trunk, leave room for

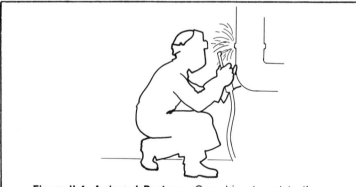

Figure II-4: Awkward Postures. Crouching to get to the proper height for a welding task is illustrated. Although this posture can be sustained for a short time without difficulty, sustained work will result in leg and back muscle fatigue and may contribute to instability in the lumbar area. Other awkward postures can result from inadequate head clearance and from working at floor or ground level.

destabilization of the vertebral column at the place where the disc may have lost some fluid and the junction is unstable. Twisting of the trunk may increase the vulnerability of the disc to rupture or accelerate facet joint subluxation and may, again, lead to a pinched nerve root.

Awkward postures often result from a designer's inadequate attention to the maintenance needs of equipment or facilities. Repair operations may have to be done under tanks or machines at sites where other equipment is in the way, so awkward postures are required to move out a motor or remove a part. In some locations head clearance has not been provided, as at the top of a production machine in a flat-roofed, low building. In warehouses, the dimensions of storage shelves are usually less than 55 inches (140 cm) high. This low head clearance is particularly awkward for the transfer of heavy items from the lowest of the shelves. Outside of work, a person may be exposed to awkward postures during car maintenance, home-improvement activities such as putting in a tile floor, and in outdoors activities including planting and weeding.

The worker may not be able to avoid some awkward postures in the workplace, but he or she should be aware of the need to take frequent "postural relief" breaks. Provision of a small "dolly" or stool to enable sitting close to the ground instead of having to crouch, or the availability of either a floor covering with good cushioning properties or a pair of knee pads for kneeling in some tasks will also improve the conditions for people with a history of backache. Unequal loads across the trunk can be counteracted in some instances by providing a firm support against which the worker can pull with the arm that is not supporting a load. This can help to even out the load on the back muscles and reduces the opportunity for a twisting motion to aggravate the unstable lower lumbar disc areas.

5. Constant Standing

Jobs that require sustained standing, especially where the standing is not broken up by periods of walking or sitting, can be difficult for people with chronic low back pain. If bending or extended reaches are also required, the problems may be

Avoid Low Back Pain Aggravators

insurmountable for some workers. Constant standing puts an unremitting load on the lumbar discs, creates back muscle fatigue from the sustained alignment of the upper and lower body during the work activities (many of which involve forward movement of the upper body), and results in orientation of the pelvis in a posture that may increase the pressure on the posterior one-third of the lumbar discs (L4 and L5, especially). If the worker is slouched forward rather than upright (but not hyperextended) the pressure on these discs will be greater. Slumping forward in a chair results in high disc pressures.

The most important workplace modifications would allow an alternation of standing and sitting during the course of the shift. Walking is also desirable for short periods. Jobs with a large amount of walking, however, may also aggravate back pain symptoms, especially if the walking includes carrying a load in only one hand. Examples of tasks where constant standing or walking may be required include those of mail carriers, guards in some institutions, kitchen cafeteria attendants, order expediters, warehouse order pickers, lathe operators, and machine control operators. Outside of work, extended periods of standing for more than one hour at a time may be needed in meal preparation and clean-up, lawn care, ironing and laundry activities, and painting, plastering, or wall-papering.

For the worker to avoid constant standing, seating should be available near the workplace such that it can be used as needed. Provision of fold-away seating is desirable, such as a "jump seat" or a seat that can be stored under the table or next to a wall until needed. If it is not available, the worker with backache should take frequent breaks to the nearest area with seating in order to relieve the stressed postural muscles. For people who work in a prescribed area and stand fairly still for much of the shift, a footrail or a small footstool, from 4 to 8 inches (10 to 20 cm) high, can retard the development of low back pain symptoms. Putting a foot on the rail will tilt the pelvis forward and relieve the pressure on the back third of the L4 and L5 discs. Rubber mats at the work station or safety shoes with good soles that are appropriate for the work and thick enough to give a cushioning effect may also be used to reduce the strain of constant standing on the feet and back.

B. SEATED WORKPLACES - POSTURES

Although many people with low back pain find relief from symptoms when they can sit down, extended sitting can in itself aggravate the symptoms. Long distance driving is an activity that can be extremely uncomfortable for a person with low back pain if the seat does not give good support to the lumbar spine. If the seat is set back, requiring full leg extension for activation of the gas, clutch, and brake pedals, back pain may result. In this section, some seated workplace characteristics are described that can aggravate low back pain symptoms by increasing the stress on the L4 and L5 discs and by decreasing the stability of the spine at this level when the disc has "flattened."

1. Lack of Foot Support

Persons with inadequate support for the feet in a seated workplace will relieve the pressure on the back of their thighs by twisting the legs around the chair supports (Figure II-5) or by supporting the feet on some part of the workbench. Both of these actions can aggravate low back pain symptoms. The leg twisting also twists the trunk somewhat and can destabilize the lumbar

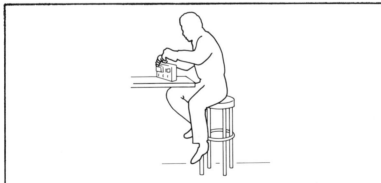

Figure II-5: Lack of Foot Support. Inadequate support for the feet can occur when a person is seated at a workbench if the chair or stool is of a fixed height and there is not enough room (height) to get the upper legs under the work surface while using the chair's footrest. The lack of foot support results in increased load on the lower spine and fatigue of the back extensor muscles if the posture must be sustained for several minutes at a time.

Avoid Low Back Pain Aggravators

spine if it is already weak due to disc flattening. Forward extension of the legs in conjunction with leaning forward to work on the workbench is somewhat like doing a straight leg sit-up. Both of these activities put a high compressive force on the L4 and L5 discs and may result in further damage to the disc casing.

There are several workplace situations where foot support can be inadequate. They include:

- A workbench surface more than 26 inches (66 cm), above the floor without a footrest. This results in adjustment of a chair beyond the point where the feet can rest comfortably on the floor.

- A chair with good height adjustability but a fixed ring footrest. When the chair seat is adjusted to 20 or 21 inches (51 or 53 cm) above the floor, the footrest is too low to keep the thighs parallel to the floor.

- A footrest in the workbench that is fixed and recessed more than 17 inches (43 cm) from the front surface of the workbench or is more than 9 inches (23 cm) above the floor, which restricts leg clearance.

Lack of an adequate footrest is seen quite frequently in offices where table or desk surfaces are 30 inches (76 cm) above the floor and chairs are adjustable from 16 to 20 inches (41 to 57 cm) above the floor. To have the person working close to elbow level on the desk, the seat would have to be at the top of its range. This brings the feet about 4-5 inches above the floor unless a footrest is available under the desk. A chair footrest is less satisfactory in office work because the worker is usually leaning forward to write or type on the desk surface. Leaning forward from the chair with one's legs near the base of the chair usually precludes use of the chair's back rest, again increasing the stress on the lower lumbar discs of the spine.

The worker can overcome the lack of a footrest by fashioning one out of an old shipping case, box, telephone books, or a pile of building materials. If footrest height is fixed instead of adjustable, a 5-inch (13 cm) height is usually preferred. The worker can also make sure to adjust his or her chair to the most appropriate height for the task being done. In general, the thighs should be parallel to the floor, not sloping downward, in order to protect the back from excessive disc pressures.

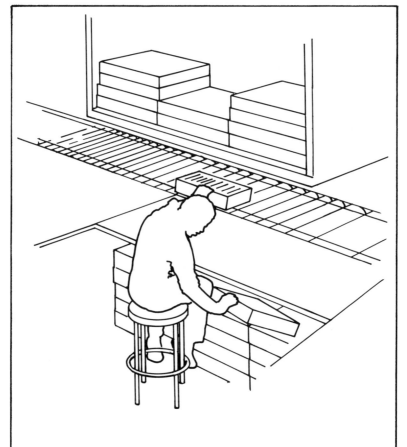

Figure II-6: Twisting in a Seated Workplace. The design of a seated workplace and the location of supplies and conveyors will affect the amount of twisting required of the worker. Supplies that are stored below the work surface can both interfere with leg clearance and cause twisting or leaning to one side when they are procured. Storage locations that are close to the work area but encourage the seated operator to get up and change posture are preferred. Too-high storage results in hyperextension of the back and should be avoided unless step stools are provided.

Avoid Low Back Pain Aggravators 31

2. Twisting - Low Supply Cupboard

Some twisting of the trunk can occur when a person has to procure or dispose of supplies from the seated posture. The design of the work station will determine how much twisting will occur. Locating the supply and disposal sites at 90 or 180 degrees away from the primary workplace assures some trunk twisting, even if a swivel chair is made available. Locating supplies or outgoing product storage areas at heights below 20 inches (51 cm) or recessed in from the front of the workplace by more than 10 inches (25 cm), results in the worker having to lean over to one side (Figure II-6). This can differentially load the spine and may aggravate back pain symptoms in people with pre-existing lumbar instability. Similarly, high shelves and ones more than 15 inches (38 cm) to the right or left of center of the worker are also likely to increase the opportunities for a worker to twist the trunk and aggravate low back pain symptoms. Two-handed lifts or force exertions in these situations are particularly difficult to do without twisting the trunk and loading the spine unevenly.

Situations where twisting of the trunk may occur while in a seated posture include the following:

- At a desk, a person turning to throw something into a wastebasket behind or to the side of the chair.

- A person accessing files at the side of the desk or reaching for a source book or paper work at the far corner of the desk or in a bookcase above the desk.

- At a seated assembly workbench, a person with stacks of trays of incoming product on the floor next to her or him; also with a stack of outgoing product for the next work station that starts on the floor.

- A person working at a seated workplace and using a pallet or skid on the floor as the source of parts or as a place to dispose of the part after this task.

- A person working at a seated workbench with supplies (like empty corrugated cases and other packaging materials) overhead in open bins. Occasional handling of these only, but they are accessed by standing up on the chair's foot ring and reaching forward and to one side.

- A two-handed lift from one side of the workbench to the other, as might occur if product comes in or goes out of the station on a conveyor that is oriented at 90 degrees to the workbench.

Similar twisting may occur where there is inadequate leg clearance, as may be the case at a kitchen sink, next to some machines, or in a standing workplace where a person is using a stool. Inability to get the knees and legs under the counter or work surface is accommodated by rotating the knees to the side and twisting the upper trunk. A table that is too low to allow thigh clearance with a fixed height chair also requires this type of trunk twisting and can aggravate low back pain symptoms.

The worker can reduce the trunk twisting by standing up to procure and dispose of supplies or parts instead of remaining seated. If there is frequent handling required (less than 2 minutes between lifts), the constant changes of posture may be annoying. The worker may be able to reorganize the workplace to keep the locations for procuring and disposing of product closer to workbench height and nearer to the main work area. Some ways of doing this include raising a pallet on 2 or 3 empty pallets, or using a "hook" or "crook" to pull a tray or container from one side closer to the workbench center. A swivel chair and/or chair with casters will permit easy changes in worker orientation if a workplace is U-shaped or requires 90 to 180 degree rotations from the main workplace. If such chairs are not available, the worker should stand up to change position. Where only occasional lifts of materials from overhead or lateral shelving are required, the worker should always stand up, since this is a way to get postural relief from constant sitting.

3. Extended Forward Reaches

An extended reach to the side of a seated workplace may result in twisting of the trunk or unequal loading of the spine that could increase the risk for low back pain. Forward reaches that are more than 15 inches (38 cm) in front of the body will require

Avoid Low Back Pain Aggravators 33

the worker to lean forward in the chair and thereby lose the benefit of any available back support. Occasional reaches are not likely to be a problem, but continuous work with extended reaches or frequent reaches that are well out of the comfortable working envelope (see Chapter 5) should be avoided. This forward bending with extended reaches is similar to forward slumping in that it puts a high compressive force on the lower lumbar discs.

Activities that can result in extended reaches include workplaces where controls are located or supplies are stored on a back panel or against a wall and the workbench is at least 24 inches (61 cm) deep. The extended reach may be to a low shelf or to a pile of trays or parts at the side of the workbench, both of which unevenly load the spine and may increase any instability at the lumbar region. Reaches forward with two hands to procure a tray, product, or part from a conveyor at the rear of a work station reduce the effectiveness of a chair's lumbar support for the person with low back pain.

The worker can avoid extended reaches by using aids to extend the reach in some instances, by standing up for occasional extended reaches, and by raising low supplies or products so that low extended reaches are not necessary. A hook on a 12-inch (30 cm) long handle with a T-grip, similar to a dock worker's hook, can be used to pull a tray off of a conveyor that runs at the same height as the work surface and to move it nearer to the worker. Provided that there is adequate leg room at the seated workplace, the worker can also pull him- or herself as close as possible to the front surface of the workbench in order to reduce the reach distance. In some workplaces a semi-circular cut-out in the workbench permits the worker to get closer to a conveyor without sacrificing a large amount of workspace.

4. Constant Sitting - Inadequate Support

As is discussed in Chapter 6 under Seating, constant sitting can aggravate low back pain symptoms as much as can constant standing. This is particularly true where chairs are not designed to give support to the lumbar spine. A person slouched forward in a chair without backrest support will have more compressive force on the lumbar discs than will the same person standing comfortably upright. Over time this force may increase the microinjuries to the disc casing and hence aggravate low back pain symptoms.

Many assembly lines are designed to maintain the flow of materials past a person's workbench so that he or she does not have to interrupt the assembly task by getting up to procure supplies or dispose of product. This results in a 2- to 4-hour period of uninterrupted sitting, which can be uncomfortable for a person with back pain. Work stations along conveyors typically tie the worker to one location and one type of posture, either sitting or standing. Other constant sitting activities include sewing machine use, word processing work, many in-process inspection tasks, some control console monitoring tasks, switchboard operation, crane operation, and long distance driving. Seat design is as critical in the vehicular setting as it is in manufacturing and office operations.

The worker can avoid aggravating back pain symptoms by adding a cushion to a chair with poor back support, purchasing a back support chair insert, or wearing an inflatable supportive vest. He or she should find opportunities to change postures frequently, and should work in the standing posture for short periods if the task does not require much bending. Upright posture is best, and slouching forward should be avoided. A brisk walk would probably be preferable to sitting down over a hot beverage during work breaks. It is also very important that the worker adjust the backrest for optimum support when possible.

C. MANUAL HANDLING TASKS

Low back pain and heavy lifting have often been causally linked, although it is more probable that they are linked primarily by the need to report back pain in heavy jobs (Rowe, 1983). If 56% of a workforce reports low back pain during their careers and 68% of those have degenerative disc disease, then up to 38% of the workforce may have repeated episodes of back pain. Those who are working in jobs that require frequent manual handling of materials will be more likely to lose time from work during these episodes than those who can control their workload and alter

Avoid Low Back Pain Aggravators

their posture. Some handling activities that can aggravate low back pain are discussed below along with suggestions for their modification.

1. Heavy Lifting

The handling of a heavy load, one that weighs more than 40 lb (18 kg) for instance, will increase the compressive force on the lower lumbar discs even if it is lifted in the most optimal manner. This compressive force is determined by the horizontal distance from the center of mass of the upper body and the load in the hands to the L4 or L5 spinal segment. The farther the person is bent forward or the load is held in front of the body, the greater is this distance, and the more work the back and hip extensor muscles must do to counteract the tendency of the body to fall forward. The heavier the load, the more work these back muscles must do to stabilize the posture, even when the object is held directly next to the body (see Chapters 5 and 7).

There are many occupational tasks that involve heavy lifting; some are easier to modify than others. For example, many foods and chemicals are packaged in 50 or 100 lb (23 or 45 kg) bags, which must be handled on and off pallets or skids. Shipping cases weighing from 50 to 75 lb (23 and 34 kg) are not unusual in industry. Seventy pounds (32 kg) is a suggested upper weight limit for some package delivery companies. Wooden pallets must be handled in some jobs, and they often weigh more than 60 lb (27 kg). In construction and maintenance tasks, a person may have to routinely lift building supplies weighing more than 50 lb (23 kg). Stock rolls or trays or bins of parts may have to be lifted into position in a machine loading task, and waste bins may have to be unloaded with similar efforts. These often weigh more than 40 lb (18 kg) each and may also be bulky.

The principal response of the worker with low back pain to these lifting tasks does not have to be a job restriction, except perhaps where heavy lifting occurs for a majority of the shift and is not easy to avoid. The use of sliding rather than lifting to move heavy objects is the best way to avoid high compressive forces on the lumbar discs. For bag handling from pallets or to machine supply hoppers, for example, a forklift truck or an adjustable-height table (levelator) can be used to bring the bag to a little above the level of the place to which it must be moved. It can then be slid off of the pallet and dropped onto the table or hopper without the full weight being lifted by the worker. In some workplaces it may be possible to provide a hoist or block and tackle to accomplish the heavier lifts; the worker with low back pain should use these. In other jobs it may not be necessary to lift the whole container if only part of its contents are needed. This would be possible in a large scale food preparation operation where only part of a bag of flour might be used to make a bread dough. Use of a scoop or smaller container to remove only the necessary material would reduce the need for lifting the heavy bag.

2. Twisting While Lifting or Pushing and Pulling

Although all manual handling training programs caution against twisting while lifting or exerting forces, people still do it because it is faster or may be the only way to accomplish the task in some workplaces. When materials have to be transferred between two locations that are oriented at 90 degrees to one another, they are often moved from one side to the other by turning the upper trunk and keeping the feet still (Figure II-7). If the object weight and size is not very great, the distance between locations is only a few feet, and if the handling frequency is low, this is probably not an activity to be concerned about in terms of low back pain aggravation. Heavier items, more frequent lifting, and more pronounced twisting can destabilize the lumbar disc area in people with degenerative disc disease. The shear forces on the L4 and L5 discs may result in subluxation of the facet joints. This can result in narrowing of the channel through which the dorsal nerve root passes, pinching it and causing very severe pain. In addition, when the trunk is twisted, the abdominal and chest muscles are not in their optimal orientation for exerting force, and they do not offer effective support and protection for the back.

Situations that result in twisting of the trunk during manual handling tasks include:

- moving an item horizontally with arms extended across a

Avoid Low Back Pain Aggravators 37

workplace, as in moving a stack of materials from left to right at the far side of the workbench.

- pulling a hand cart or truck through a corridor, using one hand and facing forward.

- working in an area where there is inadequate foot room to use a step turn. This may happen when pallets are lined up around the end of a conveyor on a fast production line (requiring the

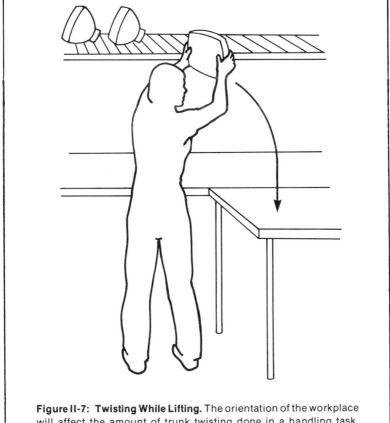

Figure II-7: Twisting While Lifting. The orientation of the workplace will affect the amount of trunk twisting done in a handling task. Removing items from a high conveyor line or shelf to a workplace located at 90 degrees to the side will often be done with a twist, especially if the frequency of lifting is high. It is preferable to design the workplace so that the lift is made totally in front of the body.

handler to lift at a frequency of 9 or more times per minute). The pallets are brought close to the conveyor in order to reduce movement time. There may not be enough space to turn the feet as product is removed to the pallets, which are usually placed at either 90 or 180 degrees to the conveyor. The handler, therefore, twists at the knees to accomplish the task.

- swinging bags or cans up from a lower level to a higher one in a warehousing or trailer unloading task. By swinging instead of lifting the bag or can, a more ballistic lift can be made and less sustained effort is required. But such a movement is made across the body rather than in front of it, and the trunk is thereby usually twisted at least 90 degrees.

- getting one's body behind an object to push it when it is being moved laterally around an obstruction. Construction tasks may require the worker to take a fixed and stable posture while exerting force with the upper trunk to locate a beam among other supports in a building frame. It is often not appropriate to make a step turn in this situation since the footing area may be limited.

- handling tasks where the terrain is rough and footing is precarious, such as on littered floors. It may be preferable to maintain a stable posture than to risk stepping and losing one's balance.

The worker with low back pain is wise to avoid trunk twisting whenever possible. The use of a step turn instead of a twist is recommended whenever stepping is appropriate. Except where it cannot be done for safety reasons, hand carts and trucks should be pushed instead of pulled through corridors in order to reduce the trunk twist associated with one-handed pulling. At conveyor palletizing stations, marks on the floor should identify the best locations for pallets so that adequate foot room for a step turn is provided. The conveyor rates should be controllable by the handler so that pace pressure doesn't make step turns too time-consuming to use. One other approach to reduce the amount of twisting in a handling task is to train the worker to pull the object to the point nearest its destination instead of picking it up earlier, where it first comes into the workplace or work site. In this way twisting can be minimized, and a footing halfway between the optimum position for either procuring or disposing of the product can be taken.

3. Uneven Lifting or Carrying

Because a person with degenerative disc disease often has instability in the lower lumbar spine, any activity that unevenly loads the spine may aggravate low back pain symptoms. A major activity in which such uneven loading may occur is one-handed carrying, especially if the object being carried is quite heavy and bulky. The weight of the object is counteracted by bending to the contralateral side, which loads the back, abdominal, and chest muscles. The shear forces on the lower lumbar discs will increase and the potential for pinching the dorsal nerve root between the bony processes of the vertebrae is greater. A similar unbalance can occur if the object being handled is not symmetrical and has more weight on one side than the other. This requires the trunk muscles to develop differential forces to keep the body in balance. Any instability of the load, as occurs if a liquid in an open container is handled, may require the trunk muscles to alter their tension suddenly in order to counteract the motion, and this too may result in instability in the lumbar region.

Occupational tasks that result in uneven loading of the spine include carrying pails of water or other liquid (Figure II-8) and carrying a heavy suitcase or bulky item with a handle at the top, such as a "portable" TV set. Furniture moving exposes handlers to many unevenly balanced loads, either because the object itself is asymmetrically weighted (as in a refrigerator and most appliances) or because the lifting and carrying task requires one hand to be higher than the other (as in taking a couch down a narrow flight of stairs with a landing). Lifting patients in a medical facility or handling pumps and other heavy equipment in a maintenance operation are other examples of uneven loading of the spine. Awkward postural requirements, such as crouching, leaning to one side, or kneeling, can also result in uneven loading of the spine as the weight is shifted from one side of the body to the other searching for a stable posture. Standing with the feet on different levels will also unevenly load the spine during a lifting task, as can two-person lifting where the handlers are not well matched in size or strength.

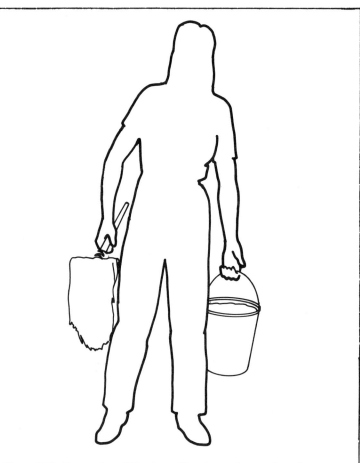

Figure II-8: Uneven Load Carriage. The cleaner is carrying a heavy bucket of water on one side of the body that is not balanced by the mop in the other hand. To keep from being pulled to the left side, she has to stabilize her posture with the back and hip extensors and with the abdominal and buttock muscles. This uneven loading of the spine increases the risk of a nerve root pinch in people with degenerative disc disease.

The person with an unstable lower back usually learns through experience that uneven loading of the spine is often associated with sharp pain. To avoid this he or she usually makes certain that loads do not become concentrated on only one side. If a suitcase is carried, it is balanced by a second suitcase or bag in the other hand; this helps to load the spine more equitably. If a force has to be exerted on one side only, the handler can stabilize his or her posture by holding on to a fixed structure with the opposite arm. In two-handed carrying tasks, the handler should try to keep the hands even and to share the load as equally as is possible. The use of straps, hand trucks, dollies, and other handling aids that permit an uneven load to be lifted or transported with both hands at the same height are also recommended (see Chapter 9).

4. Handling an Over-Sized Load

The horizontal distance from the lumbar spine to the center of a load being held in the hands will strongly influence the lumbar disc compressive and shear forces. The heavier the load and the farther its center of mass is from the spine, the more force there will be on these discs, and the more opportunity there will be for damage to them and for aggravation of low back pain symptoms. This distance will be affected by the design of the workplace or lifting task (see Extended Reaches) and by the dimensions of the items to be lifted. Bulky objects, even if they are not very heavy, extend the lever arm and put additional demands on the back and hip extensor muscles to counteract the body's tendency to fall forward. Objects that extend more than 20 inches (51 cm) in front of the body usually produce hyperextension of the back as the handler tries to reduce the load on these muscles by bringing the load closer to the lumbar spine (Figure II-9).

Some objects that are over-sized and produce awkward lifting or handling postures include:
- furniture
- trays more than 20 inches (51 cm) long and wide
- sheet materials more than 20 inches (51 cm) in length and width
- plywood sheeting
- large glass or metal plates
- bales of raw materials or waste more than 20 inches (51 cm) wide and long
- some wide stock rolls of paper, plastic, etc.

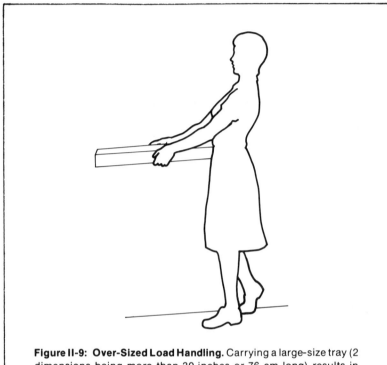

Figure II-9: Over-Sized Load Handling. Carrying a large-size tray (2 dimensions being more than 30 inches or 76 cm long) results in hyperextension of the back. The handler tries to reduce the stress on the erector spinae muscles by arching the back and moving the center of mass of the load and upper body closer to the spine. Grip is usually less stable as well because the arms have to be extended rather than the elbows lying next to the side. This instability increases the risk for losing control of the load.

Some long products (e.g., pipe) may be held in front of the body on their long dimension while being placed on a machine or in a rack. Even moderately narrow products may be over-sized in these handling tasks.

The worker with low back pain who is confronted with an oversized load often has a number of options. These include sliding the load rather then lifting it onto a transfer cart or to a pallet on a levelator in a production workplace. A rope or strap may also be used to permit the load to be grasped closer to the body if it does not have handholds. Other materials handling aids

Avoid Low Back Pain Aggravators 43

such as a dolly or hand truck may be used instead of carrying the object manually. An overhead hoist, a transfer table, or a cart could be used to support the weight of a supply roll being loaded into a machine. When multiple separate items constitute the load, such as sheets of paper, piping, metal plates, etc., the worker should restrict each lift load to 25 lb (11 kg) in order to keep the compressive and shear forces on the lumbar spin acceptable.

5. Sustained Heavy Handling or Awkward Postures

Even under the best conditions for handling heavy objects, sustained effort can produce fatigue of the back, hip, abdominal, and arm muscles, resulting in less protection of the vulnerable vertebrae in a person with degenerative disc disease. In the same manner, sustained awkward postures will selectively load some muscles, and their fatigue may make the person less able to respond to a sudden change in posture or in the balance of a load.

The unguarded move in a handling task is more likely to result in aggravation of the low back pain symptoms, as it often is accompanied by uneven loading of the spine and higher shear forces on the lumbar discs.

Sustained heavy handling tasks can be found in many warehouse and shipping areas, stockrooms, chemical or bulk food packaging areas, pallet loading operations at the end of a production machine, package delivery and bulk mail handling businesses, and ditch digging operations. The people doing these jobs spend the majority of the shift doing handling tasks, and their muscles may show some fatigue. Their overall workload can be considered heavy, requiring close to the recommended upper limit of energy expenditure for a typical shift. Jobs or tasks where sustained awkward postures may be required include many low-seam coal mining operations, some tunnel or water main construction work, some maintenance and construction tasks where clearances are tight (for example, overhead duct repairs), automobile mechanic work with extended reaches and overhead work, and construction work such as pipe fitting, where frequent bent-over postures, sustained holding, and crouching may be required.

The worker whose job requires him or her to sustain heavy lifting or awkward postures for a large part of the shift is unlikely to be able to perform that work during an attack of low back pain, and job restrictions or time lost from work usually result. By taking frequent, short breaks from the heavy work or awkward postures, usually for 1 or 2 minutes every 15 minutes of work, however, the potential for aggravating the symptoms between attacks will be less. Most people will do this intuitively unless they are paced externally by a machine, peer or supervisory pressure, or a pay incentive. The worker with degenerative disc disease should be made aware that the use of these mini-breaks will actually increase productivity by reducing the back discomfort and potential for lost time due to low back pain.

Section II: What the Worker Can Do

CHAPTER 3: KEEP MUSCLES FIT

A. MUSCLES THAT SUPPORT THE SPINE

There are four major groups of muscles that protect the lower spine by stablizing it and by counteracting high pressures on the 4th and 5th lumbar discs. These are the back extensor muscles, or erector spinae, that lie along either side of the spine, the abdominal muscles that counteract lumbar disc pressure by creating a positive pressure in the abdomen and by stabilizing the spine during turning movements, and the hip extensors and flexors, including those of the spine, buttock, and upper leg (hamstring), that provide stability to the lower spine during motions around the hips (Figure II-10).

These muscle groups act to increase the flexibility of the spine by keeping it aligned during a variety of movements such as bending forward, stretching backwards, reaching to the side, or holding an object in front of the body. The back extensors operate on very short lever arms (about 2 inches or 5 cm) and have to develop high forces to counteract the tendency of the body to fall forward when an object is lifted. The abdominal muscles are particularly important in lifting tasks because they stabilize the lower spine by fixing the trunk's posture. The increased intrabdominal pressure is in the opposite direction to the increased pressure on the L4 and L5 discs and, therefore, relieves the discs of some of the force on them. Poorly toned abdominal muscles provide less of a counteractive force and are less able to protect the spine when motions to one side are made. The hip flexors and extensors act like guy wires around the lower spine and provide stability during the full range of movements. If

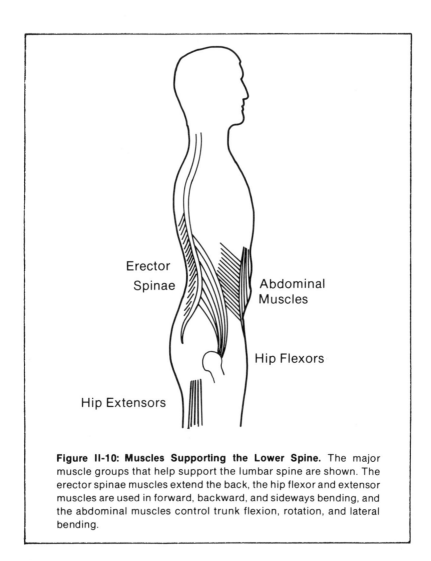

Figure II-10: Muscles Supporting the Lower Spine. The major muscle groups that help support the lumbar spine are shown. The erector spinae muscles extend the back, the hip flexor and extensor muscles are used in forward, backward, and sideways bending, and the abdominal muscles control trunk flexion, rotation, and lateral bending.

the trunk is twisted to one side, these muscles are less able to protect the spine because their force is not directly transmitted to the spine. This means that more work is done by the muscles to get the same effect of protecting the spine. As a person flexes forward to lift up an object, the muscles of the hip extensors help the back extensors keep the body from falling forward. If there is a heavy weight to be carried on one side of the body or if an object is heavier on one side, the hip flexor and erector spinae muscles work together to keep the spine balanced and stable.

B. MUSCLE STRENGTH AND FATIGUE

If the muscles of the back, abdomen, buttock, and upper leg are not kept fit they are less able to keep the spine stable as various motions are made. This can sometimes result in high compressive forces on the lumbar discs during a lifting task or during an awkward posture. The primary concern with less fit muscles, however, is not so much the peak forces required in certain tasks but the muscles' inability to sustain moderate workloads for extended periods. For example, a muscle with less capacity because of a lack of exercise will fatigue faster at the same workload than will a fit one. This is particularly important for tasks where the required posture is leaning forward or to one side or where an object has to be held or carried for more than a few seconds.

Figure II-11 shows the relationship between the percent of muscle strength used (% MVC) and the length of time it can be exerted continuously (in minutes). The higher the capacity (MVC, or maximum voluntary contraction strength), the lower % MVC any given task will be. Thus, if a person has a grip strength of 100 pounds (or about 45 kg), a 50-pound (23 kg) object held in that hand uses 50% of grip strength. If the grip capacity is only 75 pounds (34 kg), however, the same object uses 67% of grip strength. The 50% MVC load can be held for 1 minute continuously, whereas the 67% MVC load can be held for only 45 seconds before muscle fatigue occurs. Thus, the person with less capacity will have to take more frequent recovery breaks (see Chapter 10), and this may affect his or her productivity in a heavy job. A similar situation occurs for the back muscles. Their capacity for a given task will depend on the biomechanics of the posture or the lifting situation. The force exerted by the back extensor muscles, for example, will be acting on a 2-inch (5 cm) lever. That will have to counteract the object weight on a lever from the spine to the center of mass of the body and the object being lifted (see Chapter 5). The farther the body is from the upright posture and the heavier the load, the higher the percent of back extensor maximum strength required, and the sooner fatigue will occur. Keeping the back muscles well-toned will reduce the risk of overexertion by increasing their strength and making each task a lower percent of that maximum value.

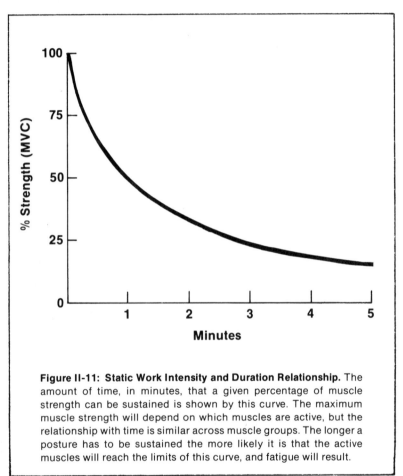

Figure II-11: Static Work Intensity and Duration Relationship. The amount of time, in minutes, that a given percentage of muscle strength can be sustained is shown by this curve. The maximum muscle strength will depend on which muscles are active, but the relationship with time is similar across muscle groups. The longer a posture has to be sustained the more likely it is that the active muscles will reach the limits of this curve, and fatigue will result.

C. EXERCISES TO KEEP THESE MUSCLES FIT

There are a number of exercises that can be used to stretch, tone, and strengthen the four groups of muscles that protect the lower back. The ones summarized below are suggested because they can be done equally well by people with healthy backs and by people who have a history of low back pain.

Keep Muscles Fit 49

1. Bent-Knees Abdominal Curl (Figure II-12) - Lie on your back with your knees bent and heels flat on the floor. Clasp your hands behind your head. Slowly raise your head, shoulders, and upper trunk off of the floor on a count of 3. Then, slowly lower yourself again on a count of 3. Breathe out as you come up. Repeat 5 to 10 times initially, increasing the number to 20 times later as you become better conditioned.

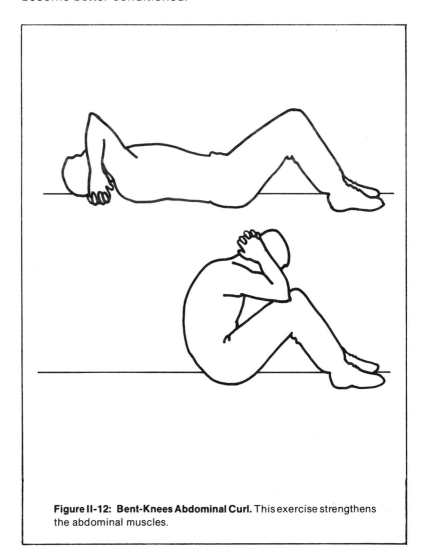

Figure II-12: Bent-Knees Abdominal Curl. This exercise strengthens the abdominal muscles.

2. Leg Pull (Figure II-13a) - Lie on your back with your knees bent and your heels flat on the floor. Bring one knee up to your chest and clasp it with your hands. Keep your head on the floor. Hold the knee up for 10 seconds, then return the leg to its bent knee position and repeat the stretch with the other leg. Repeat the cycle 3 times for each leg initially and increase to 5 times later. Then raise both knees to the chest at once and hold for a count of 10 before relaxing again. Repeat this 3 times.

3. Cross Over Stretch (Figure II-13b) - Lie on your back with straight legs. Bend your right knee and cross it over your left leg. Put your left hand on your right knee and stretch your right arm to the side. Turn your head to look at your right arm, keeping your shoulder and head on the ground. Pull down on your right knee and hold it for a count of 10. Then relax and repeat it again. Change legs and do the same stretch twice on the left leg.

4. Whole Body Stretch (Figure II-13c) - While standing, clasp your hands over your head and turn your palms upward. Your feet should be a shoulders' breadth apart. Slowly stretch your arms over your head looking straight ahead and keeping your hands together. Do not hold your breath or go up on your toes. Repeat 5 times initially and up to 10 times later on.

5. Side Slides (Figure II-13d) - Standing with your feet a shoulders' breadth apart, press your right hand against the outside of your right thigh and slowly slide it down, leaning to the right with your trunk. Come back to an upright posture and then repeat the slide with the left arm and leg. Repeat the cycle 5 times initially and up to 10 times later on.

If these exercises are done every other day and at a moderate level, the back, buttocks, hamstring, and abdominal muscles will be toned. The suggested number of repetitions should not be exceeded, especially during the initial conditioning stages.

Muscle spasm is a common outcome when a nerve root is pinched in the lower spine. The pinched nerve causes increased activity of the motor neurons which increase back muscle contraction strength, and this further increases the pain in a positive feedback loop. One has to break the cycle by stretching out the muscle or by reducing the pinch on the nerve root to stop

Keep Muscles Fit 51

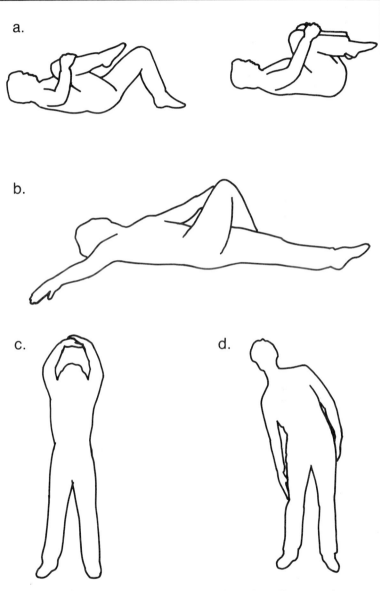

Figure II-13: Four Back Strenghtening Exercises. Four exercises that help to strengthen the hip flexors ("a" and "b"), the lateral trunk muscles ("b" and "d"), and the trunk extensor muscles ("c") are illustrated. See the text for instructions.

the muscles from going into spasm. The best approach is to curl the legs up to your chest to take the pressure off the nerve root by opening up the space between the vertebrae. With the chin down and your arms down at your sides, the stretch on the back muscles should reduce the spasm as well as reduce the trigger from the pinched nerve. Lying on the floor with the lower legs on a chair seat usually gives relief if a nerve pinch/muscle spasm is caught early enough.

Some recent research suggests that whole body exercises may be preferable to specific exercises for the back as a way of preventing low back pain episodes. Whole body muscle toning can improve the way in which one works at any job since there is less probability that any muscle will limit the performance of a task. If the whole body exercise program includes back exercises, then it may be preferable as long as exercises that may be difficult for a person with low back instability (such as back arching and some straight leg stretching exercises) are not required. Any exercise is better than none, but too much exercise at high intensity or of extended duration is not advisable, especially when starting or resuming an exercise program.

Section II: What the Worker Can Do

CHAPTER 4: LIFT SAFELY

Manual handling tasks are associated with a high incidence of occupational low back pain reports. One corrective approach used for many years has been to train people how to lift safely so that the risk of overexertion is reduced. Defining safe lifting then becomes the challenge, since what people do in the workplace is not always consistent with what is considered the best lifting practice by safety and ergonomics specialists.

A. SAFE LIFTING AND LOW BACK PAIN

Despite a strong emphasis on training programs for at least 30 years, there has not been a concomitant decrease in the incidence of reports of low back pain in industry. As Rowe (1983) has suggested, the low back pain problem associated with manual handling tasks may be related more to the need to report the pain when doing heavy or repeated lifting or force exertion than to a problem with the way the object is lifted. The person with degenerative disc disease may benefit from learning safe lifting techniques, but the application of those techniques may not reduce the probability that he or she will have an episode of low back pain on the job.

Safe lifting techniques can be expected to reduce overexertion injuries of the arm and shoulder muscles. A reduction in strains and sprains can be expected for a period of 3 to 6 months after a lifting training program because people are more aware of good body mechanics and how to use their muscles effectively during handling tasks. As with most training programs, however, the benefits will begin to "wear off" after six months. The major points will have to be reinforced at least once a year, preferably in a new format, in order to maintain the lowered incidence of reported strains and sprains.

Despite the difficulty of showing that low back pain problems are significantly different before or after lifting training, information about safe lifting techniques should be provided at the workplace. Explanations of body mechanics, patterns of work that increase or decrease the potential for muscle fatigue, and special techniques developed by people who lift for a living (such as dock workers, furniture movers, and shipping dock handlers) can help others develop appropriate methods for their handling tasks.

B. GENERAL LIFTING GUIDELINES

There has been considerable discussion over the past 10-15 years about the appropriate way to teach lifting. The method used for many years suggested stereotyped postures with the legs always bent, back straight, chin in, and with the legs doing the lifting. Several researchers have noted that few people when left to their own devices use this technique - except when the object to be lifted is very heavy. Many workers handle objects weighing up to 30 pounds by using a modified derrick lift; the knees are not used to do the lifting, but one leg is stretched out to counterbalance the load on the spine as the object is raised from the floor to a table. Other forms of dynamic or free-style lifting, most of which involve a combination of knee and back bending, have also been observed. Most researchers agree that the stereotyped lifting technique may not be optimal for every worker. The guidelines given below (and in Figure II-14) are general ones that apply across different types of lifts, whether they are done free-style or in a more stereotyped lifting posture.

1. Do Not Twist While Lifting

This is perhaps the most critical factor in the design of lifting tasks and in their execution. The muscles that support the spine and keep the discs and vertebrae aligned even if there has been some loss of fluid from the disc have been enumerated in Chapter 3. Twisting will reduce their effectiveness and increase the rate at which they fatigue, especially if the object being lifted is heavy.

Lift Safely

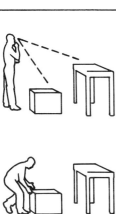
a. Plan the Lift

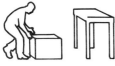
b. Determine the Best Lifting Technique

c. Get a Secure Grip

d. Pull the Load In Close To Your Body

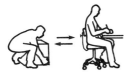
e. Alternate Lifting and Light Work Tasks

Figure II-14: Guidelines for Lifting. Five guidelines for performing manual lifting tasks are illustrated. See the text for further discussion.

The orientation of the workplace will affect the person's tendency to twist as will the amount of foot clearance and the rate at which the lifts must be made. Chapter 5 discusses design factors that can influence the amount of twisting done during lifting tasks.

2. Plan the Lift

Sizing up the load and determining how it will be lifted and where it will be placed is one way of avoiding overexertion injuries. An unplanned lift may result in the handler having to support the load longer than is necessary. This can produce local muscle fatigue that may increase as the shift proceeds and limit the worker's ability to sustain the work for a full 8 hours. The closer the weight of the object is to the capacity of the weakest muscle groups involved in the lift, the faster these muscle groups will fatigue, and the more opportunity there is for a muscle overexertion injury to occur. The relationship between duration and intensity of effort shown in Figure II-10 illustrates the impact of extended holding times, as might occur in unplanned lifts, on available strength.

One aspect of planning a lift is to determine if it is too heavy or bulky for one person to handle. By assessing the situation first instead of starting directly in on the lift, one can decide if a handling aid, a cart, or another person is needed to move the object.

3. Determine the Best Lifting Technique

The size, weight, and location of the lift, the frequency at which it must be repeated, and the duration of continuous lifting are all factors that will help determine the best lifting technique. Compact objects (see Chapter 9) lend themselves to better lifting postures than do bulky objects, and heavy objects require more use of the legs for lifting then do light ones. Lifting frequency and duration should be considered when deciding on the lifting technique, because an awkward posture may become a limiting factor in extended lifting tasks. Calisthenics associated with lifting up the body every time an object is lifted may also limit a person's capacity for a lifting task if the legs are bent for each lift. However, a "derrick" (or stoop) lift (Figure II-15) is not recom-

Lift Safely

4. Take a Secure Grip on the Object Being Handled

The hand is the interface between the object being lifted and the person; how secure the grip is will determine how safe the lift will be. If the object has handholds (see Chapter 9), a good power grip can be used and stability is less of a problem. Many of the objects to be lifted, however, are not equipped with handholds. Examples of these include shipping cases, bulk materials in bags, sheet materials such as plywood, and raw materials such as metals. The grip type will depend on the configuration of the load. Wherever possible, a power or ledge support grip (see Figure II-14 "c") should be used rather than a pinch grip, which has only 25% of the strength of a power grip.

If a handler's grip is not secure there are at least two potential concerns relating to back problems. The first is that the person may lose control of the load while handling it and may take an awkward posture or lose his or her stable foot position while trying to get the load back into control. This can result in a slip or trip accident which may aggravate a back problem. The second potential problem is if a pinch grip is used and the hand and arm muscles fatigue before the lift is completed. The need to readjust the load to use different muscles can result in overexertion of the arm or shoulder muscles or twisting of the trunk providing there is no place to set the object down first. Poor grip stability, then, can contribute to low back pain symptoms if handholds are not available and the duration of holding the object is more than a few seconds.

5. Pull the Load in Close to Your Body

Lift location determines both the amount of compressive force on the lower lumbar spine and the strength available (i.e., which muscles) for making the lift. The discussion of work location in Chapter 5 explains why this factor is so important. Every lifting technique emphasizes the need to get the load close to the body to prevent excessive stress on the back and to make the strongest muscles of the arms available to hold the load. If the load can be held close to the body, the grip is usually more stable and the shoulder muscles do not limit the duration of holding. In addition, a person can walk normally without having to hyperextend the back in order to counteract the forward pull of the load.

Some lifting situations make it difficult to keep the object close to the body because the handler cannot bend his or her knees due to an obstruction. Objects that are handled near the floor and that are too large to fit comfortably between the legs during lifting will cause the lift to occur at a greater horizontal distance from the spine than is desirable. In some of these situations a lifting aid or a second person may be needed to reduce the risk of overexerting the muscles or putting excessive pressures on the lumbar discs.

6. Alternate Lifting Tasks with Lighter Work

Heavy lifting is not usually sustained because people recognize that their muscles are fatiguing and find ways to take breaks to rest the muscles. Sustained moderately heavy lifting tasks are more common, often found at the ends of conveyor lines where materials are loaded or unloaded at a fixed rate. These can become problem tasks, especially if an awkward posture such as leaning to one side, bending forward, or twisting is incorporated in the way the lifting is done. The design of lifting tasks and the need to provide adequate recovery time in repetitive lifting jobs are discussed in Chapters 7 and 10, and some suggestions for ways to structure jobs where repetitive lifting is done for a majority of the shift are included in Chapter 11. The general guideline for job design is to provide alternate tasks that do not heavily stress the same muscles. These lighter tasks allow the active muscles to recover and are alternated with the lifting tasks throughout the shift.

C. OTHER MANUAL HANDLING TECHNIQUES

Not all objects are "lifted" in the workplace; but in choosing guidelines for handling materials manually one has to assume that one person's "lower" may become another person's "lift." Lowering takes less energy to perform but the general guidelines given in "B" above are still appropriate for these tasks. Two other types of handling are discussed below: two-person lifting and sliding or pushing.

Lift Safely 61

1. Two-Person Lifting

There is a general assumption that if one person should not be making a lift, two people can do it. Although this may be appropriate for bulky loads that are not very heavy, it is not necessarily appropriate for heavy lifting. Even if a team of handlers is well-matched in terms of their body size, strengths, and work capacities, they cannot always perfectly share a load when handling it together. Thus, it is not true that two people can lift twice as much weight as one person can. Some suggestions for determining when two-person lifting is most appropriate are given below:

a) When an object to be handled has two dimensions that are more than 30 inches (76 cm), even if it is very light, two people can probably handle it more safely than can one.

b) If a lift is being done very infrequently and the object exceeds the guidelines for one-person lifting but is not more than 50% heavier than the one person lifting weight limit, it can probably be safely handled by two people.

c) If the object to be handled is very long (pipe, conduit) and is awkward for one person to balance without hyperextending the back, a two-person lift is recommended.

d) If items, such as bags, are handled frequently and for extended durations (more than one hour continuously), total lifting time and local muscle fatigue can be reduced by having two people handle them together.

2. Sliding and Pushing

Local muscle fatigue can become a problem when an object is handled frequently for extended periods. Inadequate time for the active muscles to recover between exertions will cause a build-up of fatigue, and the opportunity for an overexertion injury to occur will be greater. One approach to reduce this fatigue is to reduce the amount of effort for each transfer of the product by not actually lifting it. Designing the workplace so the object can be transferred using a push, pull, or slide can reduce the muscle work and make the total workload more acceptable as well. Guidelines for the amount of force to be exerted and for the design of handling tasks to permit the use of sliding are included in Chapters 7 and 8.

Section III: How the Workplace Can Be Improved

Chapter 5: Work Location - Heights and Distances

Chapter 6: Seating

Chapter 7: Design of Manual Handling Tasks

Chapter 8: Special Workplace Aids for People with Low Back Pain

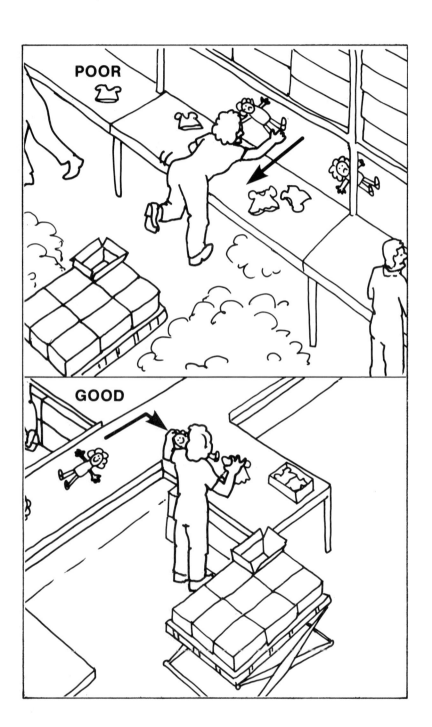

Section III:
How the Workplace Can Be Improved 5

Even if the worker tries to minimize over-exertion on the job, workplace design factors can contribute to his or her low back pain symptoms. These include work heights and reaches that are inappropriate for sustained work, poor seating, and repetitive lifting tasks done in workplaces where unnecessary effort is built into the job. Identification of these workplace problems and suggestions of ways to overcome them by better design and worker accommodations are covered in this section.

CHAPTER 5: WORK LOCATION - HEIGHTS AND DISTANCES

Where the hands are located when a task is performed and how closely the body posture conforms to an upright alignment of the spine will determine the stress on the lower back. Body mechanics, or biomechanics, can be used to analyze the direct, shear, and rotation (torque) forces on the lower spine and the muscle work required to keep it aligned. The compressive, shear, and rotation forces are important contributors to small tears in the disc casing that can result in fluid loss from the disc and instability in the L4-L5 (fourth and fifth lumbar) vertebral column. The demands on the hip flexor and extensor, erector spinae, and abdominal muscles to keep the spine aligned are greater when this instability is present (see Chapter 3). The consequences of their failure to keep the spine aligned can be a very painful compressed nerve root. In this chapter some discussion of the biomechanical stresses on the back is presented, and guidelines for the design of working heights, reach distances, and workplace orientation are given.

A. LOCATION AND BODY MECHANICS

The spinal column is designed to support the weight of the body and forms curves at two locations, at the cervical region (below the head) and at the lumbar region in the lower back. These curves are towards the ventral (or belly) side. When a person is standing upright the center of mass of the body is centered over the skeleton and ankles so minimal muscle effort is required. If the person reaches forward or to the side, the muscles of the trunk have to do extra work in order to counteract the tendency of the body to follow the arm in that direction. Alternatively, the person has to realign other parts of the body, such as one leg, to reverse the forward fall and to reestablish the center of mass over the skeleton. A teeter-totter analogy simplifies the mechanics. Assume that child #1 weighs 50 pounds (23 kg) and child #2 weighs 25 pounds (11.5 kg). The length of the teeter-totter board is 20 feet (6 meters). If the board is pivoted around its center, child #2 will never be able to get child #1 off of the ground because the balance point requires an equation of force times distance on each side. At the board's midpoint:

Child #1		Child #2
(50 lb) (10 ft)	vs	(25 lb) (10 ft)
500	vs	250

If the teeter-totter board is set so that child #1 is only 5 feet (1.5 m) from the pivot point, child #2 will be 15 feet (4.6 m) from that point and can lift and hold the heavier child off the ground.

Child #1		Child #2
(50 lb) (5 ft)	vs	(25 lb) (15 ft)
250	vs	375

If the two children are to be equally balanced, the distance from child #1 to the pivot point should be 6.7 feet (2.0 m) and child #2 should be 13.3 feet (4.1 m) from this point.

Work Location-Heights and Distances

The trunk extensor muscles, or erector spinae, are the primary muscles involved in keeping the spine upright. If one leans forward, the erector spinae are activated to pull back on the trunk. The weight of the upper body becomes the equivalent of one of the children on the teeter-totter. The work of the erector spinae muscles to counteract the upper body motion is equivalent to the other child, measured as force rather than weight. The lever arms, or distances, on which the forces work are: the distance from the spine to the body's center of mass when the person leans forward, which is the force arm (upper body mass that has to be counteracted); and the distance from the insertion of the erector spinae muscles to the same point on the spine, which is the resistance arm (muscle work to counteract the forward lean). The resistance arm is about 2 inches (5 cm) long, and is fixed by one's anatomy. Unlike the children on the teeter-totter, then, the resistance lever arm can not change, so the work of the erector spinae muscles is directly proportional to the horizontal distance from the spine to the center of mass of the body or to the center of mass of the body plus the weight of an object held in the hands or carried on the trunk. The farther that weight is from the ankles, the more work the back extensor muscles have to do and the faster they will fatigue. An example of the impact of horizontal distance on compressive forces on the spine is shown in Figure III-1.

The forward bending moment has to be counteracted by activity of the erector spinae muscles and this force is transmitted to the lower spine. The posterior third of the fourth and fifth lumbar discs (L4 and L5) are most "vulnerable" to these forces as they form the "S-shaped" curve of the lower spine.

Shear and rotational forces on the lumbar discs will be created if the upper body is moved to one side, as in bending to one side or reaching across the body, or if the trunk is rotated to one side even if the body is still upright. This unequal loading of the spine puts the back and hip extensor muscles at biomechanical disadvantage. The forces they develop are not fully transmitted to the spine because of the altered orientation of the force arm due to the twist. This would be somewhat analogous to putting a bend at one end of the teeter-totter. Because the force is not in line with the pivot point, the board's stability will be greatly

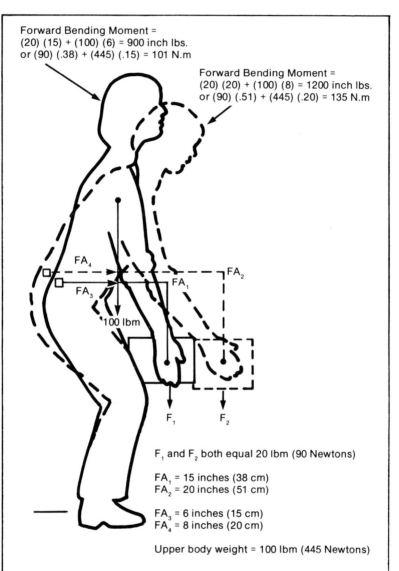

Figure III-1: Load Location and Forward Bending Moment. The forward bending moment is a function of the weight of an object held in front of the body and the weight of the body as the handler bends forward. The moment is the sum of these weights times their force arms or levers. FA_1 and FA_2 are the distances from the spine to the center of the load and FA_3 and FA_4 are the distances from the spine to the center of mass of the upper body.

Work Location-Heights and Distances 69

reduced. In the case of the spine, the trunk and hip flexor muscles will have to work harder to apply the same force to the force arm, and they will, therefore, be more subject to fatigue.

When an activity requires high reaches or overhead work, the spine is arched backwards or hyperextended. This motion mechanically compresses the posterior third of the L4 and L5 discs especially, and puts the erector spinae muscles at a disadvantage because they are no longer stretched for optimal tension development. Repeated hyperextension of the back may increase the opportunities for disc flattening in persons with degenerative disc disease, thereby reducing stability in the lower spine.

B. WORKING HEIGHTS AND REACHES

Work surface height will determine the amount of stress on the back and shoulder muscles for work that is done by people of very different body sizes. The most comfortable working heights are at or around elbow height. If forces are applied, the work surface should be below elbow height. If fine visual attention is needed, the surface should be higher. A too low work surface results in static loading of the back extensor muscles or the legs because the worker has to lean forward, bend over, or bend the knees to get into the right posture for the work. A too high work surface requires the worker to elevate the elbows to do the task; this puts a static load on the shoulder muscles that can result in their early fatigue.

Anthropometric data of the elbow heights of people standing upright (Figure III-2) suggest that a standing work surface should be between 35 and 41 inches (89 and 104 cm) above the floor, the lower value for tasks where force exertion is needed and the upper value for visually-demanding work. For seated work the elbow height is measured relative to seat height. It assumes that the seat height can be adjusted to meet the work surface height needs. Elbow heights range from 7 to 12 inches above the seat. Seated work surface heights can be varied from 25 to 32 inches (64 to 81 cm) above the floor providing a footrest is available for people with shorter legs (see Figure III-3).

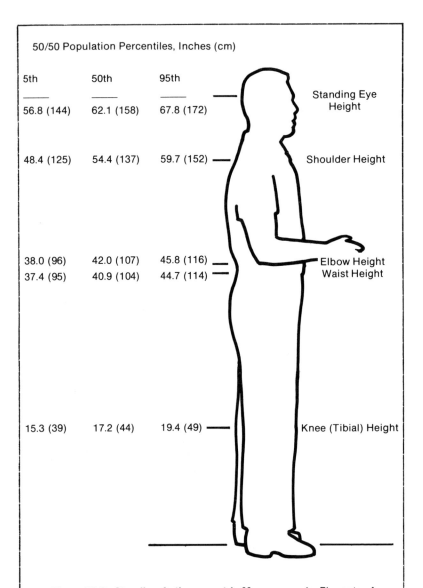

Figure III-2: Standing Anthropometric Measurements. Five sets of values are shown for 5th (small), 50th (average), and 95th (large) percentile heights for a mixed population (men and women). The values are given in inches and centimeters. These are useful in determining appropriate heights for the design of standing workplaces.

Work Location-Heights and Distances

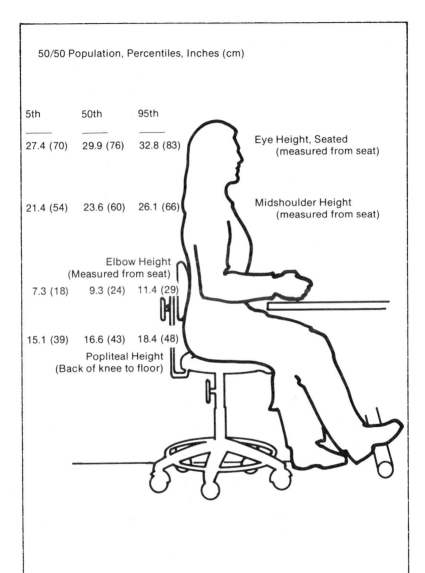

Figure III-3: Seated Anthropometric Measurements. Four sets of anthropometric measurements that are useful for seated workplace design are shown. The values are for the 5th, 50th and 95th percentile heights based on a mixed population of men and women. All of the heights except popliteal height are measured from the seat pan, not the floor.

Standing forward reach capability is a function of arm length and of the height at which the reach is made. The range of motion of the shoulder in moving the arm up and down in front of the body is in an arc with the greatest forward reach available at shoulder level. As the arm moves above shoulder level it loses forward reach capability, falling from 22 inches to 15 inches (56 to 38 cm) as it moves from 54 to 72 inches (137 to 183 cm) above the floor. At 80 inches (203 cm) above the floor the forward reach is less than 5 inches (13 cm). Below shoulder level the forward reach is also less. Many tasks are done at these heights, and the worker has to lean forward or bend down to get the additional reach capability. At elbow height, for example, most people have only about 15 to 18 inches (38 to 46 cm) of forward reach, and at mid-thigh height (about 30 inches, or 76 cm) their forward reach has decreased to 5 inches (13 cm).

If the reach is not directly in front of the body, but is done more towards one side, an additional 3 to 5 inches (8 to 13 cm) of forward reach may be lost. If two arms are needed instead of one to reach an item, forward reach is about 2 inches (5 cm) less in front of the body. It is even more severely reduced if the reach is more than 25 inches (64 cm) to one side of the center of the body.

A general guideline based on the reach and height inter- actions suggests that work surface heights should be kept between 35 and 41 inches (89 and 104 cm) for standing tasks whenever possible. Forward reach requirements should be kept within about 15 inches (38 cm) of the front of the body in order to reduce the need for bending to extend the reach (Figure III-4). Lower and higher work heights are commonly found and are associated with either back or shoulder muscle fatigue in many people. Overhead assembly or repair work, as in installing duct work or working under a car in a repair shop, should recognize that more than 5 inches (13 cm) of forward reach will be difficult for smaller workers.

For seated work the same forward reach arc applies; the farther to the side or the higher the reach is, the closer the object to be reached must be. Forward reaches of 15 inches (38 cm) at the work surface (Figure III-5) and no more than 10 inches (25 cm) forward at 25 inches (64 cm) above the work surface are

Work Location—Heights and Distances

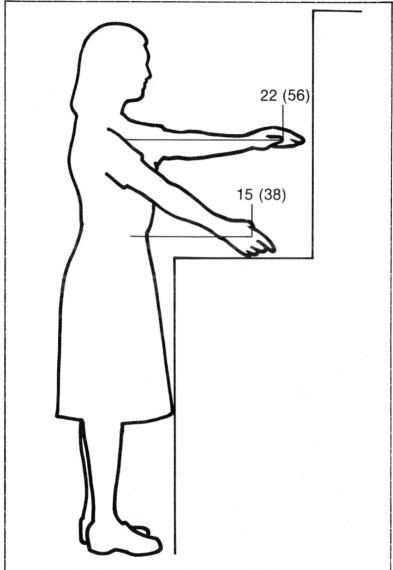

Figure III-4: Standing Forward Reach Capability. The forward reach capability of a small person (5th percentile functional arm reach from the front of the body) in a standing workplace is shown at 35 and 50 inches (89 and 127 cm) above the floor. The guideline of keeping forward reaches within 15 inches (38 cm) of the front of the body is developed from this anthropometric data.

recommended. If the reaches exceed these values, the worker will have to lean forward and may lose backrest support. This could result in an aggravation of symptoms for a person with back pain who has to sit for a majority of the shift.

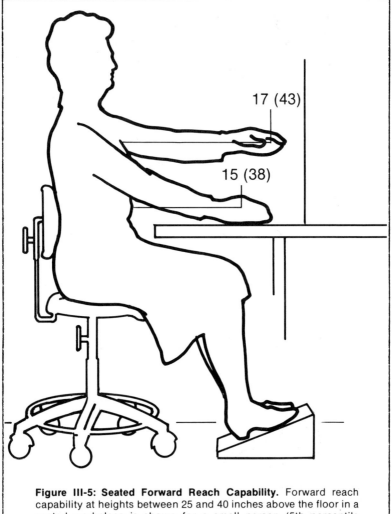

Figure III-5: Seated Forward Reach Capability. Forward reach capability at heights between 25 and 40 inches above the floor in a seated workplace is shown for a small person (5th percentile functional arm reach from the front of the body). The 15 inches (38 cm) forward reach guideline for design of seated work tasks is based on this anthropometric data.

Work Location-Heights and Distances

Reaches below the work surface at a seated workplace are of concern because forward reach is very limited (to a few inches). The worker will often have to twist to reach an object that has to be handled or operated. Repeated movements below the work surface may also result in rubbing the trunk on the chair's backrest and can produce local skin abrasions. In general, materials, items, or equipment that have to be reached or activated frequently should be located near the work surface and within the recommended forward reach dimensions given above. Materials that have to be accessed infrequently might better be placed where the operator has to get up to obtain them. This would assure some postural adjustment in an otherwise predominantly seated task.

C. ORIENTATION OF THE WORKPLACE

The way the workplace is designed will influence how much turning or twisting a person has to do to accomplish the work. The illustration at the beginning of Section III illustrates two designs, one where the work is done in a 180-degree arc and other where the work is kept within a 90-degree arc. In the first example, the operator has to turn 180 degrees from the conveyor to the pallet for each cycle. This 180-degree rotation in each direction can increase the shear and rotational forces on the lower lumbar discs and will reduce the effectiveness of the abdominal and hip flexor muscles in supporting the lower spine.

Orienting the workplace to keep the movement pattern within a 90-degree arc reduces the opportunities for extreme twisting and reduces the movement time as well; this makes it possible to complete more assemblies per shift if the operation is self-paced. In the example in Figure III-6, the 90-degree arc is created by placing the packing work surface perpendicular to the supply table. The worker can reach the incoming product better and load it directly into the packing boxes, which can be at a lower level. The packed boxes can be placed on the pallet in another, separate, 90 degree turn. The supply table can be used as temporary on-line storage to relieve the time pressure of the conveyor's delivery of product.

These changes in the orientation of the workplace relative to the conveyor line and the pallet are intended to make it more difficult for the worker to twist and put shear forces on the lower spine. Other designs reduce extended reaches by making a cut-out (semi-circular) in the work surface so the worker can access materials that would otherwise be outside of a comfortable reach. These designs can be used both in standing and sitting workplaces. This approach reduces the potential for fatigue of the extensor muscles of the back by keeping the body more upright during work.

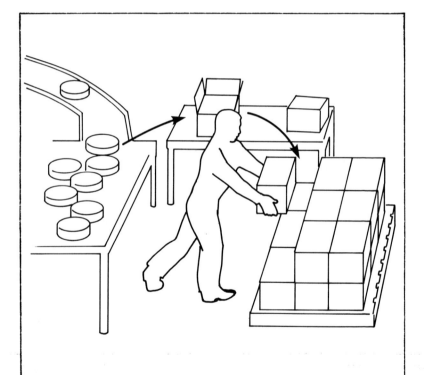

Figure III-6: Workplace Orientation in a Packing Task. An example is shown of a workplace design that permits two 90 degree turns to be made in a packing cycle. The product arrives via a conveyor to a supply table, is packed at a second, lower table. The cases are then transferred to the pallet after several have been filled. This reduces the need for twisting a full 180 degrees as could occur if the packing is done on the supply table.

Work Location-Heights and Distances

When materials, such as boxes or parts, have to be stored in and around the workplace, the guidelines for height, distance, and weight in lifting tasks (see Chapter 7) should be followed. The orientation of the supplies or parts should be such that they can be moved without twisting or hyperextending the back and are not so low that the legs interfere with lifting them. These limitations suggest that storage areas should be from 20 to 55 inches (51 to 140 cm) above the floor, whenever possible.

Section III: How the Workplace Can Be Improved

CHAPTER 6: SEATING

There is a common policy of taking people who have low back pain out of standing jobs and putting them in jobs where they can sit for the majority of the shift. This policy is probably based on the observation that if one stands all day, backache often results. However, sitting all day can be equally hard on the back, especially if the chair being used is not well designed or if there are not supplementary aids such as footrest available. In this chapter some information about chairs and how they influence the stability of the low back is presented. An approach to selecting a chair for the workplace is presented in Appendix B.

A. TYPES OF WORKPLACES - STANDING, SITTING, AND SIT/STAND

The decision about whether a job will be a seated or a standing one is made primarily on the basis of the type of work to be done. Although it is considered preferable to provide seating, if possible, many tasks make it necessary to keep the worker on his or her feet for a majority of the shift. Some of the job demands that make a standing workplace more suitable than a sitting one are:

1) When work has to be done over distances that exceed the comfortable arm reach envelope (about 15 inches or 38 cm on either side of the body).

2) When work is done on a moving part or conveyor and the worker has to move along with the part.

79

3) When the work is spread out over several parts of a machine or in a storage area.

4) When the height of the work above the floor is variable and some of it cannot be easily reached from a seated posture.

5) When heavy weights are handled or large forces must be exerted.

6) When the visual needs make a seated posture inappropriate, either because of difficulty in seeing something on the line or because one has to move around to get the best angle to view a display.

In the above job conditions a standing workplace will be preferable to a seated one; but during periods when the worker is waiting for others or monitoring the equipment, a chair or support stool could be used for postural relief of the back. The opportunity to sit even for short periods should reduce the stress on the back from continuous standing and should, therefore, reduce the complaints from those with recurrent low back pain.

Sitting workplaces are more often observed in light assembly tasks, inspection stations, and in other tasks done primarily with the arms and hands, including typing, data entry and retrieval on computer terminals, and other record keeping. If a person is in a job where he or she is kept sitting for the majority of the shift, the chair provided in the workplace should be carefully chosen to give good postural support to the back. These chair characteristics are detailed below. Jobs that do not give a person the chance to get up and walk around fairly regularly are often found to be associated with complaints of low back pain from people who already have symptoms. Examples of these types of tasks include work where everything is delivered to the seated workplace and finished product is removed by someone else or by a conveyor. The worker does not have to get up to procure new supplies or dispose of the completed work, so he or she remains seated for 2 hours continuously. Workplaces at conveyors where assemblies, inspection, or other tasks are done on a part as it comes past the worker in the seated station may also make the worker "captive" to the chair. This is especially true if the conveyor heights are most appropriate for seated work and the tasks are not easy to perform in a standing posture.

Sit/stand workplaces have been recommended for many years by ergonomics and human factors specialists because the option for either sitting or standing provides postural relief for the back. Designing a good sit/stand workplace is not very easy, however, because a work height that is good for a standing workplace is too high for a seated workplace. Simply adjusting the chair upwards to get the worker's elbows up above the work surface is not satisfactory because it is difficult to get on and off of a chair when its seat is adjusted to more than 21 inches (53 cm) above the floor. In view of this difficulty, special supports or sit-stools have been recommended. In general, these provide a seat that the worker can lean against while the legs remain in a mostly standing posture. The support provides some relief for the back; the feet can be rested, too, if there is a standby break in the work. These support stools are not as readily available as are chairs, but they have appeared in production furniture advertisements more frequently over the past few years. Many of the designs first came from Scandinavian countries.

B. CHAIR DESIGN

The design of chairs for use in offices or production areas should incorporate several common features (Figure III-7). For production or office workers who are seated for a large part of the shift, well-designed chairs are necessary to avoid back pain, to provide good support for the trunk and legs, and to reduce forms of discomfort, such as result from pressure on the back of the thigh, that might contribute to reduced individual productivity.

1. Chair Seat Height Adjustability

A good chair must be adjustable in height so it can optimize the working height for a person's hands. The lower limit of adjustability should be low enough so that people with short lower legs can place their feet on the floor and still keep their thighs parallel to the floor while seated. The upper height adjustment should be to at least a level where people with very long lower legs can sit without having their knees well above their hips. For this reason, chairs that adjust between 15 and 22 (38 and

Working With Backache

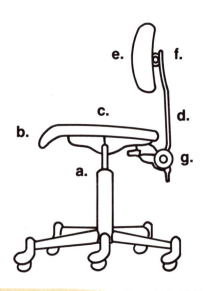

a. Seat Height Adjustability	From 15 to 22 inches (38 to 56 cm)
b. Seat Width	17 to 19 inches (43 to 48 cm)
c. Seat Depth (or Length)	17 inches (43 cm)
d. Seat Slope	5-10 degrees up (towards the front)
Chair Backrest	
e. Size	6-9 inches (15-23 cm) high 12-14 inches (30-36 cm) wide
f. Movement Up and Down	7 to 10 inches (18-25 cm) above the seat
g. Movement In and Out	12 to 17 inches (30-43 cm) from the front of the seat

Figure III-7: Recommended Seating Design. The recommended chair height adjustability, seat dimensions, and backrest design are summarized. See the text for discussions of the recommendations.

Seating 83

56 cm) inches above the floor (seat pan to floor distance) are recommended. Higher adjustability may be useful for situations where footrests are built into the workplace and where work surface heights are fixed at greater than 30 inches (76 cm) above the floor in a seated workplace.

2. Chair Seat Width

If a chair is to be used comfortably by a large proportion of the workforce, it should be wide enough to give good support to the buttocks but not so wide that sliding on and off is difficult. If the chair has arms, the inside distance between the arm rests will have to be wide enough to accommodate a large person's hip breadth plus any winter clothing worn. This would be about 19 inches (48 cm). If there are no arm rests or lateral limits of comfort (see below), then a width of 17 inches (43 cm) should be adequate.

Chair design that produces an "edge" at the limits of the seat's width causes discomfort because the force per unit area on the buttocks is considerably greater on the edge than on the seat pan. This can limit lateral mobility and postural adjustments in the chair and increase back discomfort because of the restriction. Such edges are more commonly seen in molded plastic chairs than in fabric-covered seating. They should be avoided in making selections of cafeteria, conference room, or auditorium chairs whose chief virture is that they stack well.

3. Chair Seat Length or Depth

Recent surveys of home and office chairs indicate that the chair seat depth (front to back of the seat) is often greater than the distance between the back and the back of the knee (buttocks to popliteal distance) of many people. If this is true, then people sitting on those chairs often have to slide forward in order to be able to put their feet on the floor. By sliding forward they may not be able to get the benefit of the backrest (discussed below), so there is a greater possibility of developing back pain symptoms during extended sitting. To accommodate the upper leg length of most people, chair seat depth should not exceed 17 inches (43 cm). If the depth is much less than this, however, people with very long upper legs will have inadequate leg support. Thus, a seat depth of 17 inches (43 cm) is probably optimal. This dimension interacts with the height adjustment characteristics of the chair. A chair that does not adjust below 18 inches (46 cm), for instance, should have a seat depth of not more than 17 inches. The drag on the back and upper leg will become excessively fatiguing and painful if the person with shorter legs cannot reach the floor with his or her feet and also cannot use the chair's back support. A footrest will relieve this discomfort somewhat, but seat depth should also be specified to improve seated comfort.

4. Chair Seat Slope

Recent discussions of chair seat slope have provided recommendations to slope it 5 to 15 degrees up or to design it 45 degrees down and have the worker sit and kneel simultaneously to relieve the back. The usual recommendation is to slope the seat pan up slightly (about 5-10 degrees) so the front of the seat is about 1 inch (2.5 cm) higher than its back. The seat height adjustability is measured from the seat's front surface. Too much upward slope of the seat restricts leg movements forward for postural relief; the edge of the chair becomes a pressure point for the underside of the upper leg. A rounded edge with padding is preferable to a plastic or metal edge. A continuation of the chair's seat beyond the turned edge assures that a sharp edge will not produce discomfort when the legs are brought back alongside the chair base during activities where the worker has to lean forward.

The recent introduction of seating that angles the seat forward and provides rest points for the knees and ankles is based on the theory that tilting the pelvis forward will reduce the stress on the lower spine and provide more comfortable seating over long periods. Such seating appears to be best in tasks where the worker does not have to lean forward to write or to do a task requiring force exertion. The weight must be evenly spread between the buttocks, knees, and ankles to avoid symptoms of "housemaid's knee" or sore ankles in extended sitting on these chairs.

5. Chair Backrest

The backrest of a chair should be large enough to give support to the spine without interfering with sideways motions. It should be adjustable up and down and in and out, or it should be formed to provide lumbar (lower spine) and upper thoracic (below the shoulders) support. The usual recommendation for the size of an adjustable height backrest is from 6 to 9 inches (15-23 cm) high and 12 to 14 inches (30-36 cm) wide. It should be able to move from 7 to 10 inches (18-25 cm) above the seat height in order to fit most people's need for lumbar support. It should also be able to adjust in and out from 12 to 17 inches (30-43 cm) from the front of the seat. This will provide support to the back when a person is leaning forward about 5 inches (13 cm). Without such horizontal adjustability, the worker who performs a job with extended forward reaches at a seated workplace gets little benefit from a backrest (Figure III-8).

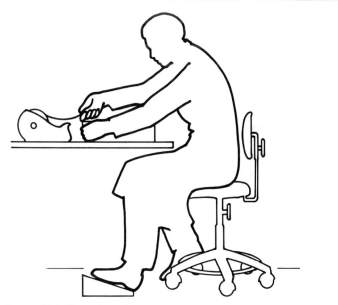

Figure III-8: Work Location and Backrest Utilization in a Seated Workplace. A seated workplace job involving a wrapping task requires the worker to lean forward. He or she loses back support because the backrest does not easily move forward. If this task is done for several minutes continuously, symptoms can occur in people with recurrent low back pain.

More recently chairs are available that are molded or covered with fabric to support the whole back, and they are adjustable as a unit (Figure III-9). Either the back follows the worker as he or she leans forward because it is springloaded, or the worker uses a push button adjust to bring the backrest forward as needed. The design of the backrest in these chairs will determine how effective they are in reducing back stress during prolonged seating. If the major support for the spine is near the shoulder blades, the pressure on the L5 (fifth lumbar) disc will not be reduced as much as it will if there is support both there and in the lumbar region. If the backrest is sloped backward about 15 degrees, the compressive force on the lumbar disc will be less than if it is upright. The backrest in a molded chair or in an "office chair" must be designed in view of the need for support at two places on the spine. Adjustability that allows the worker to benefit from the backrest when he or she is leaning forward in the chair (Figure III-9) is also desirable.

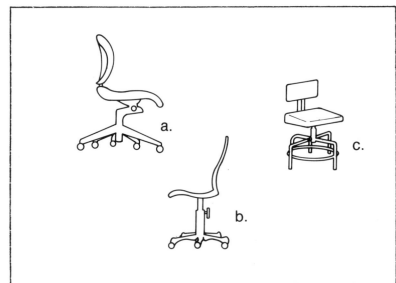

Figure III-9: Molded and Tubular Chair Design. Examples of a molded office chair with fabric covering ("a") and of two inexpensive molded ("b") and tubular ("c") chairs that are typically used in production or assembly areas are illustrated. Selection of these types of chairs should emphasize the backrest design characteristics shown here.

Seating 87

6. Other Characteristics - Swivel, Support, Covering

Chairs that are used in workplaces where workers do not have opportunities to get up or to change posture should be stable, should move easily to the side so twisting is not required of the worker, and should be covered with a material that "breathes" so that localized sweating does not occur. Most industrial chairs have 4 or 5 legs to provide stability against tipping. The 5-legged version is recommended if the seated worker has to reach for objects that are outside of his or her comfortable reach distance (usually more than 15 inches, or 38 cm, away). As body weight is shifted to one side, upwards or downwards, the 5 legs provide a stable base and reduce the chance that the chair will tilt with the worker.

Since it is likely that a person working at a seated workplace will occasionally, if not frequently, have to get supplies, parts, or tools at locations to one side of the body or the other, it is important to provide swivel capability in the workplace chair. If the chair will swivel, and if there is adequate leg clearance, then the needed items can be procured without twisting the upper body. Such twisting is a major aggravator of low back pain symptoms and should be avoided.

The fabrics used to cover a workplace chair are often chosen according to aesthetic, cost, or durability considerations. Although these factors are important, one should also consider the worker's comfort. How well the material breathes and whether prolonged sitting will result in stickiness and sweating has a significant effect on worker comfort. The choice of a molded chair with or without additional padding may be best resolved by considering how long the worker has to stay in it. Plastic, unperforated coverings, and other fabrics that do not breathe should not be used in workplaces where extended sitting is required and where seasonal temperatures may exceed the upper comfort zone level of 78 degrees F (25 degrees C).

The decision about which chair should be used at a seated place is influenced by the cost, durability, appearance, and perceived importance of the chair. The design factors described above will influence how comfortable the chair is for the worker

Working With Backache

and whether low back pain symptoms are more likely to be aggravated with extended sitting. Using the guidelines for chair selection found in Appendix B, one can try to optimize the chair for the workplace and job in order to reduce the potential for back pain problems.

C. FOOTRESTS AND ARMRESTS

To provide optimal comfort in a seated workplace it is advisable to provide an adjustable footrest as well as an adjustable chair. The footrest will give the worker more options for adjusting his or her height relative to the work surface. If the work surface is high, the chair can be adjusted to a higher part of its range so the work is near elbow height. As long as the footrest is available to support the feet of people with shorter legs, the higher workplace can be used comfortably by most workers.

Footrests are available as plates that can be adjusted in height and in degree of tilt. A surface that is at least 16 by 12 inches (41 by 30 cm) in length and width should hold both feet comfortably, and it should tilt up from the horizontal surface no more than 30 degrees (see Figure III-5). Height adjustability in 2-inch (5 cm) increments is recommended. Styrofoam packaging material, phone books, and shipping cases have been used as makeshift footrests in some places. These are better than no footrest, but they do not tilt to provide the best comfort for the ankles in the seated posture.

A footrest can also be built into the workplace station, either as part of the bench structure or as part of the chair (see Figure III-3). The main disadvantage of chair or workbench footrests is that they tend to be in fixed locations and do not offer the possibility of postural adjustments. Footrest rings on chairs are sometimes not adjustable in height, so the ring can only be used when the chair is in the low part of its height range. As the chair goes up, the footrest no longer keeps the thighs parallel to the floor, and discomfort in the low back area is more likely to result.

Armrests are useful aids in jobs involving, for example, prolonged assembly or inspection tasks. The armrests may be on the chair when monitoring or light work is done while the worker

Seating

sits back in the chair. They should not run the full depth of the seat, however, because they may make it difficult to pull the chair up to the workplace. If the arms do not fit under the work surface when the chair is near the top of its height adjustment, the worker may not be able to get close enough to read the video display or paperwork at the workplace. Then he or she may have to lean forward, losing the chair's back support and potentially incurring back muscle fatigue and pain.

Armrests that are attached to the work surface and can be adjusted in many directions have been used in some fine dexterity assembly work or in other work done primarily with the hands and fingers. These armrests reduce the static muscle loading of the shoulder and arm muscles and reduce the potential for tremor to occur in the hands. The most important attributes to look for in armrests are:

1. Adjustability - including distance, angle, and tilt.

2. Padding for comfort - using fabric or materials that breathe and don't cause heat accumulation and sweating.

3. No sharp edges - so there is no discomfort caused by high force per unit area on the skin on the inside of the forearm as it lies on the armrest.

4. Ease of adjustment - an ability to change the direction of the arm rest by exerting additional force on it or using a simple fastener, like a wing nut, to reset the orientation.

For further information on chair, footrest, and armrest design, see Appendix B.

Section III: How the Workplace Can Be Improved

CHAPTER 7: DESIGN OF MANUAL HANDLING TASKS

Work involving lifting, lowering, pushing, and pulling of materials is often associated with reports of low back pain in industry. Some possible reasons for that association are discussed in this section. Guidelines for the design of occasional and frequent lifting tasks and force exertions are also given.

A. ASSOCIATION OF MANUAL HANDLING AND LOW BACK PAIN

Studies of the incidence of low back pain are complicated by the variety of ways in which the data are collected. A questionnaire that asks if people "have ever had" low back pain gets quite different information than a search of medical records to see if the same people "have ever reported" low back pain. If the question is further refined to "Have you ever lost time from work for low back pain?" the numbers become still lower. A similar problem occurs in trying to define the relationship between manual lifting and low back pain. One has to classify the lifting or handling requirements in a way that identifies the potential risk to the lumbar discs or to back, arm, or shoulder muscles. At extreme lift locations or heavy weights, for example, this risk is reasonably easy to define. In the center of the continuum, however, the definition is less clear, and this makes it difficult to attribute the incidence of back problems to specific lifting conditions.

Studies from Eastman Kodak Company, the University of Michigan, and Liberty Mutual have identified the following relationships between manual handling and low back pain:

1) People who work in heavy jobs have more need to report low back pain symptoms than do people in lighter jobs (Rowe).

2) Lifting that puts high compressive forces on the L4 and L5 discs (more than 650 kg) is associated with twice the average number of low back pain reports (Chaffin and Park).

3) People who perform lifting tasks requiring muscle strengths that are above the acceptable levels for 75% of the working population report three times more low back pain (Snook).

On the basis of this evidence, it is advisable to examine the design of manual handling tasks and to try to design them so the disc compressive forces are not too high, the strengths required will accommodate of least 75% of the potential workforce in terms of "acceptable" lifting conditions, and the postures do not further aggravate low back problems because of twisting or uneven loading of the spine.

B. HANDLING LOCATION

The biomechanics of postures and loads on the lumbar spine have been discussed in Chapter 5. When an object is lifted, the center of mass of the body and the load is pulled forward (longer force arm) and the back extensor muscles have to do additional work to keep the body from falling forward. In the teeter-totter analogy, adding the load to one child's end means that the other child has either to increase the load on the opposite end or to lengthen the lever in order to balance the board. The back's muscle lever is fixed, so this option is not available; the only way the increased load can be counteracted is to change the amount of force exerted by the extensor muscles. This analysis assumes that body postural adjustments, such as moving one leg to help stabilize the load, cannot be done. Such a situation may exist, for example, if a load is lifted from a low position or over an obstruction (Figure III-10).

The amount of strength available to lift an object will depend on where it has to be handled from, where it is going, and how one has to get it there. Figures III-11 and III-12 show the relative isometric (static) pull strengths available at 12 locations above

Design of Manual Handling Tasks

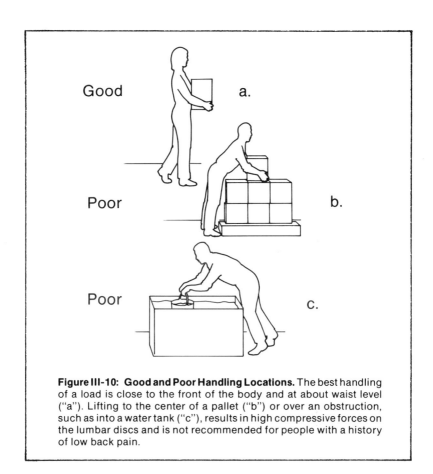

Figure III-10: Good and Poor Handling Locations. The best handling of a load is close to the front of the body and at about waist level ("a"). Lifting to the center of a pallet ("b") or over an obstruction, such as into a water tank ("c"), results in high compressive forces on the lumbar discs and is not recommended for people with a history of low back pain.

the floor and in front of the ankles for men and women. Although dynamic lifting strength is less than static pull strength, the relationships between the amount of strength that can be made available at each location should be similar. The table shows the most static pull strength at the point where the load is 13 inches (33 cm) above the floor and within 7 inches (17 cm) in front of the ankles (horizontal distance). As the tray is pulled upward at 32, 52, 72, or 74 inches (81, 132, 180, or 185 cm) above the floor, muscle strength is reduced significantly. This reduction is related to the dropping out of the leg, back, and upper arm muscles and increased reliance on the weaker forearm and shoulder muscles. At each height, there is an additional decrement in strength if the tray is located farther in front of the ankles. This is a lengthening of the force arm, increasing the load on the back. It also results in more the force being generated by shoulder instead of upper arm, trunk, and leg muscles.

The loss of strength with location is greater for the females than for the males. This is probably related to the average differences in body size and, therefore, lever lengths for the extended horizontal pulls; it is also explained by the available muscle groups dropping out faster at each of the vertical distances. Average knee, waist, and shoulder heights for males and females are indicated on the drawings to the right of the relative strength tables in Figures III-11 and III-12.

The reduction in strength as an object is handled higher or farther in front of the body means that any weight becomes a greater percentage of strength in these positions. A 20-pound (9 kg) box may represent 20% of maximum voluntary lift strength at 13 inches (33 cm) above the ground and 7 inches (18 cm) in front of the ankles. If it has to be lifted to a shelf that is 52 inches (183 cm) above the floor and can still be kept as close to the body, it can take up to 80% of the strength available at that level. The short time the load has to be held will probably make that lift acceptable, but repeated lifts at frequencies above 6 per minute could result in muscle fatigue and a further reduction in lifting capacity.

Although the lower heights for lifting are where more muscles are available, the stress on the lower back at these heights is usually greater. The person with degenerative disc disease will be most comfortable lifting in a range from 32 to 50 inches (81 to 127 cm) above the floor. This is the range where the lift can be made by the upper arm muscles, aided by slightly bending the knees at the lower end and without having to hyperextend the back at the upper end. Figure III-13 illustrates the poor and good ranges for the design of lifting tasks for the majority of the workforce. Lifts that are less than 10 inches (25 cm) or more than 50 inches (127 cm) above the floor are not recommended, especially in repetitive lifting tasks. In all circumstances, the load should be carried as close to the body as is possible, preferably within 10 inches (25 cm) of the ankles (as measured horizontally).

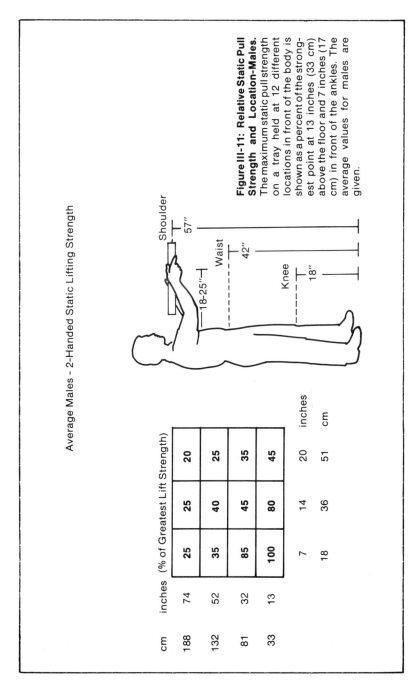

Figure III-11: **Relative Static Pull Strength and Location-Males.** The maximum static pull strength on a tray held at 12 different locations in front of the body is shown as a percent of the strongest point at 13 inches (33 cm) above the floor and 7 inches (17 cm) in front of the ankles. The average values for males are given.

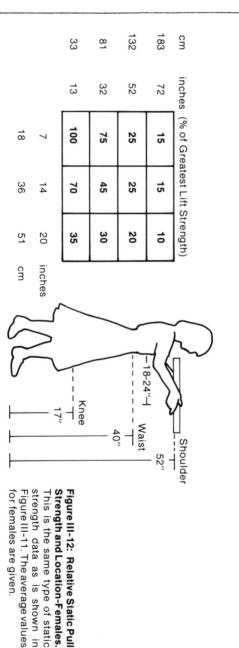

Average Females - 2-Handed Static Lifting Strength

inches (% of Greatest Lift Strength)				
72	15	15	10	
52	25	25	20	
32	75	45	30	
13	100	70	35	
	7	14	20	inches
	18	36	51	cm

cm: 183, 132, 81, 33

Figure III-12: Relative Static Pull Strength and Location-Females. This is the same type of static strength data as is shown in Figure III-11. The average values for females are given.

Design of Manual Handling Tasks

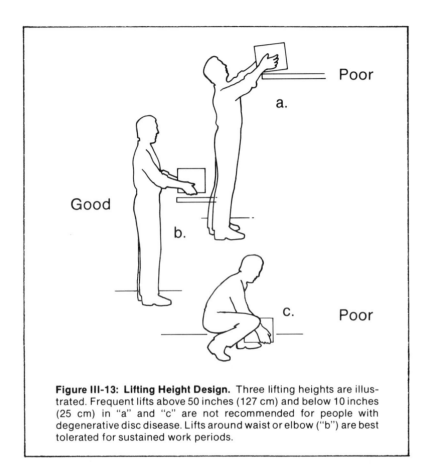

Figure III-13: Lifting Height Design. Three lifting heights are illustrated. Frequent lifts above 50 inches (127 cm) and below 10 inches (25 cm) in "a" and "c" are not recommended for people with degenerative disc disease. Lifts around waist or elbow ("b") are best tolerated for sustained work periods.

Location of the lift should also consider the need to avoid unequal loading of the spine and twisting. If the object to be lifted is located behind an obstruction, or if the handler has to take an awkward posture because of limited foot clearance at the workplace, twisting or uneven handling may result and increase the shear and rotational forces on the lower back. The design of large storage containers, for example, makes awkward lifts likely when trying to remove parts from the bottom. Unless a side can be broken down or a walk-in side is provided to allow easier access to the bin, the handler ends up doing a "derrick lift" to procure the lowest part. This type of lifting is particularly difficult and inappropriate for people with degenerative disc disease.

C. LIFTING GUIDELINES TO REDUCE LOW BACK PAIN AGGRAVATION

There are three major factors to consider when choosing appropriate lifting guidelines for people with a history of low back problems. Lift location is one of these and has been discussed above. The second factor is the amount of weight that can be lifted. This will be determined by muscle strength and is highly influenced by lift location and the load's configuration. The weight also will influence the amount of force on the lumbar discs, so biomechanical considerations as well as strength measures are of interest. The third factor relates to workload and local muscle fatigue, both of which are influenced by the rate of lifting and the duration of continuous work. In this section guidelines for occasional and frequent lifting are presented.

1. Occasional Lifts - The NIOSH Manual Lifting Guidelines

Figure III-14 illustrates the guidelines for lifting that have been developed by a committee for the National Institute for Occupational Safety and Health. This graph is applicable only for lifts done less frequently than one lift every 2 to 5 minutes and where the lifting range is between 20 to 40 inches above the floor. They assume 2-handed lifts in the sagittal plane (in front of body), a compact load, good handholds, good posture, and smooth lifting in a temperate environment. The weight of the object to be lifted is shown on the vertical axis and the horizontal distance from the ankles (or spine) is given on the horizontal axis. Two curves are shown. One marks the upper limit of the zone of recommended lifting task design and is called the Action Limit (AL). The other marks the upper limit of weight considered safe for people to lift even if they have been specially trained and selected and is called the Maximum Permissible Limit (MPL).

The design of lifting tasks in the Acceptable Lifting Conditions zone will assure that at least 75% of the women and 99% of the men will have the strength needed to make the lifts. At the MPL, only 25% of the males and 1% of the females have the required strengths. The recommendation of the NIOSH Guideline is to train or select people for jobs including lifts in the

Design of Manual Handling Tasks

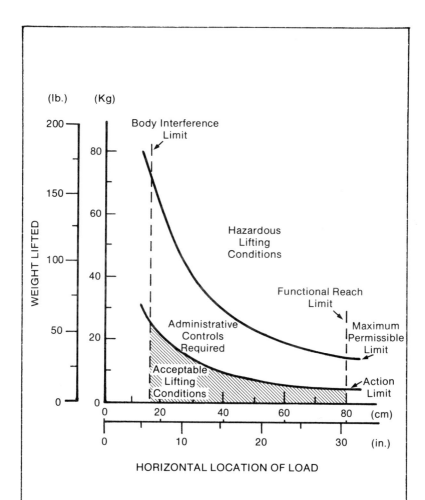

Figure III-14: NIOSH Manual Lifting Guidelines. The weights that can be lifted at different horizontal locations in front of the ankles are shown by three zones. The Acceptable Lifting Conditions Zone is where manual handling tasks should be designed to be suitable for most people. The guidelines were developed by a committee for the National Institute for Occupational Safety and Health. See the text for further explanation of the use of these guidelines.

Administrative Controls Required Zone because many people will find the lifts difficult.

The graph in Figure III-14 can be used in several ways. If one knows the weight of the load, it is possible to estimate what percentage of the workforce may find a given lift acceptable or possible. By defining the horizontal location of the load when it is lifted and finding the intersection point between that value and the weight, a point is obtained that can be evaluated relative to the AL and MPL lines. If the point falls below the AL, then more than 75% of the women and 99% of the men are accommodated. If it falls above the MPL, less than 25% of the men and 1% of the women are accommodated. Between these two curves the point can be related to the distance it is from either extreme. The percentage of the population accommodated can then be interpolated. If the point falls halfway between the 2 curves, for instance, then 99 - (0.5) (99-25), or 62% will determine what percent of the men will be able to do the job safely. For the women the calculation is 75 - (0.5) (75-1) or 38% who can do it safely.

A second way to use the guidelines is to take a given location of a lift and figure out the heaviest object that can be handled by most people (AL or below) at the workplace. The point of interest is fixed by the AL curve as it intersects the horizontal distance value. The weight is read off of the vertical axis at that point. Similarly, one can specify the object weight and use the guideline to decide when a handling aid would be advisable because of an awkward horizontal lift requirement.

Since not all lifts are done at 20-40 inches above the floor, the NIOSH Manual Lifting Guide also includes formulae for calculating the AL and MPL weight limits for other lift locations. These are as follows:

English Units:
$Al(lb) = 90(6/H) (1 - .01 | V-30 |) (0.7 + 3/D)$

Metric Units:
$Al(kg) = 40(15/H) (1 - .004 | V-75 |) (0.7 + 7.5/D)$

H is the horizontal distance factor when the load is picked up. It is in inches or centimeters.

V is the vertical height factor or the height at which the load is picked up, and is also in inches or centimeters. The difference between 30 inches (76 cm) and the actual height is treated as an absolute value ("|V-30|"). This means that the sign is disregarded and 20 inches (51 cm) up is considered equivalent to 20 inches (51 cm) down as a factor influencing lifting task design.

D is the vertical lift distance from beginning to end of the lift. If it is less than 10 inches (25 cm), it is assumed equal to 10 inches. It should generally be the difference between the starting and ending V values.

The MPL values are obtained by multiplying the AL value by 3.

The NIOSH guidelines are primarily useful for determining how to design lifting tasks and whether a specific task is difficult for a large percent of the workforce. There are situations when the weights calculated for the AL do not make sense. These most often occur when the occasional lifts do not meet the assumptions mentioned above and some other factor, such as pinch grip strength or pressure on a joint, is more limiting than the back, arm, and shoulder muscle strengths. Whenever a handling task is being evaluated, one should look carefully to see if there is a limiting muscle group or a condition that makes the task difficult to perform. With that situation in mind, one can calculate an AL and MPL, but those values should not be used for design until the task is simulated to see if they are appropriate.

2. Frequent Lifts

If lifting is done more than once every 2 to 5 minutes there is potential for build-up in local muscle fatigue and for the total workload to limit the acceptable weight to be handled. Repeated exertions, even if they only last a few seconds, need recovery time to restore the energy supply of the muscles. The amount of strength required to do a task and the number of muscle groups that can be applied to the work will determine the percent of capacity used by any one muscle group. The higher that value, the longer it will take to regenerate the energy supplies for the next effort. The closer those efforts follow one another, the more opportunity there is for the energy supply to fall below its optimal level and, with time, the more potential there is for the heavily loaded muscles to fatigue.

Lifting frequencies that exceed 6 per minute appear to have increased potential for local muscle fatigue to develop. Since many lifts take only 2-3 seconds to perform, the recovery time after each lift is about 7 seconds. For high strength requirement tasks, the ratio of work to recovery time should be at least 1 to 3 to avoid cumulative fatigue. While 6 lifts per minute will be within this guideline for short duration lifts, higher lifting frequencies will not be. Because fatigue builds with time, frequent breaks in the lifting task to do some other, less physically-demanding, work will permit some additional recovery to occur. The duration of lifting tasks that are done more than once every 2 minutes should be chosen to reduce the chances for significant fatigue to develop in the active muscles.

The work of repetitive lifting puts demands on the cardiovascular system (heart and blood vessels) to deliver enough oxygen and nutrients to keep the muscles working. The longer that activity level has to be sustained, the more stress there is on the cardiovascular system. Acceptable levels of aerobic work vary according to the number of minutes or hours they have to be sustained before a lighter activity or recovery period is provided. Figure III-15 illustrates the relationship between intensity and duration for aerobic work. By definition, maximum aerobic work capacity for the task can be sustained for 6 minutes before exhaustion sets in. One hour of continuous lifting would be the upper limit for a task that takes 50% of aerobic capacity, but it would take at least an hour to recover from the hour of work. If a repetitive lifting task is done for a full 8-hour shift, the work should take no more than one-third of the aerobic work capacity for these muscles.

Figure III-16 shows the relationship between weight handled and lifting frequency based on data from psychophysical and physiological studies. The psychophysical studies ask the workers to adjust weight to a value that would be "acceptable" to

Design of Manual Handling Tasks

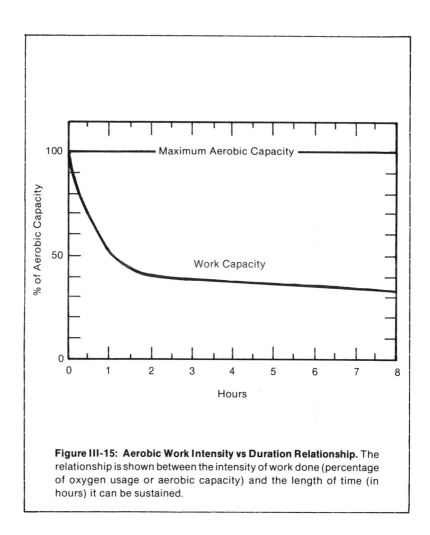

Figure III-15: Aerobic Work Intensity vs Duration Relationship. The relationship is shown between the intensity of work done (percentage of oxygen usage or aerobic capacity) and the length of time (in hours) it can be sustained.

lift at the frequency indicated. These studies were based on 40 minutes of lifting and extrapolated by the worker involved to an 8-hour day. The physiological studies are based on measurements of the heart rate and energy demands of the lifting tasks; they determine the guideline values for sustained work. These combined data suggest that at frequencies from 1 to 6 lifts per minute, the total energy requirements of the job are within most people's capabilities providing the loads are kept below 40 lb (18 kg). The higher the frequency of lifting, the lower the weight should be to reduce the potential for local muscle fatigue or for excessive workload in terms of energy requirements. To simplify, one can generalize as follows:

a. At lifting rates below 1 per minute the psychophysical study data best describe the potential stress of the job. The NIOSH Manual Lifting Guide graph and formula can be used to calculate the AL (Action Limit) for these jobs.

b. At lifting rates from 1 per minute to 6 per minute the acceptable weights are affected by the length of time the effort has to be sustained in each lift and the amount of recovery time left before the next lift. The psychophysical data shown in Figure III-16 can generally be used to determine the acceptable lifting weights in this range.

c. At lifting rates above 6 per minute, total workload must also be considered. Data from studies of the metabolic and cardiovascular demands of lifting tasks can help to determine what the acceptable weights and frequencies will be. Total workload can be controlled by limiting the time of continuous lifting to 20 minutes or less, the higher frequency lifting being done for very short continuous periods. In self-paced operations these limitations are often worked into the job. In machine-paced operations, the design of the line may make it difficult to limit the periods of continuous lifting; it is those jobs where overexertion injuries are more frequently seen.

d. Objects that weigh more than 33 lb (15 kg) should be handled by sliding rather than lifting at rates of 6 per minute or more.

D. FORCE EXERTION GUIDELINES

It has been recommended that sliding rather than lifting is preferable for repetitive handling tasks in order to reduce the potential for local muscle fatigue. The amount of force that can be exerted depends on the location of the object, how accessible it is and whether one can get behind or in front of it, and on one's posture during the push or pull. Relative muscle strengths available for pulling up on a tray at several locations in front of the

Design of Manual Handling Tasks

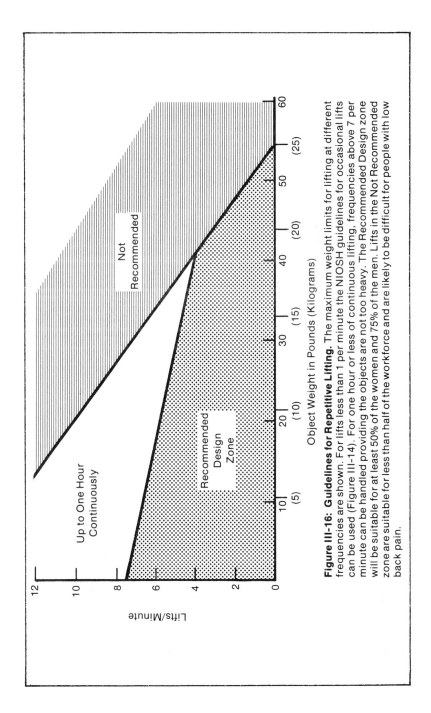

Figure III-16: Guidelines for Repetitive Lifting. The maximum weight limits for lifting at different frequencies are shown. For lifts less than 1 per minute the NIOSH guidelines for occasional lifts can be used (Figure III-14). For one hour or less of continuous lifting, frequencies above 7 per minute can be handled providing the objects are not too heavy. The Recommended Design zone will be suitable for at least 50% of the women and 75% of the men. Lifts in the Not Recommended zone are suitable for less than half of the workforce and are likely to be difficult for people with low back pain.

Force Conditions	Maximum Force for Design	
	Pounds	Newtons
Whole Body, Standing		
Forward Push, Truck Handling		
Initial Force	50	220
Sustained for 1 Minute	25	110
Emergency Stop	80	355
Pull In, Waist Level	55	245
Pull Up from Floor Level	125	555
Pull Up from 20 Inches (51 cm) Height	70	310
Kneeling	40	180
Upper Body, Standing		
Pull Up, Waist Height	55	245
Pull Up, Shoulder Height, Arms Extended	30	135
Boost Up, Shoulder Height	60	265
Pull Down from Overhead	100	445
Push Down, Waist Level	75	335
Lateral Push Across Body	15	65
Seated		
Forward Push, Waist Height		
Near	30	135
Arms Extended	25	110
Pull Upward, Elbow Height	25	110
Pull In, Waist Height, Near	20	90
Lateral Push Overhead	10	45
Lateral or Transverse Push Across Body	20	90
Foot Pedal Activation	90	400

Table III-1: Maximum Force Application Recommendations. Data on the maximum static force levels for design of handling tasks is summarized for different muscle groups. The values shown accommodate half of the female workforce and most of the male workforce. It is assumed that these forces will be exerted for only a few seconds unless otherwise noted.

Design of Manual Handling Tasks

body have been given in Figures III-11 and III-12 and are discussed in Chapter 5. Table III-1 summarizes some data on recommended upper limits for force exertion tasks done while standing or sitting and when having the whole body strength or just a few muscles to apply to the object.

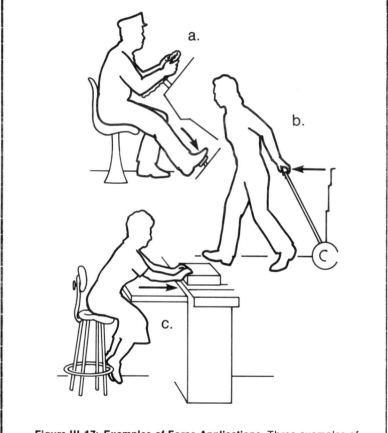

Figure III-17: Examples of Force Applications. Three examples of forces applied by different muscle groups are given. In "a" the foot pedal force is developed primarily by the lower leg, whereas the cart handling task in "b" involves whole body pulling where the most strength is available. In task "c" the assembler pushes the product onto the conveyor and often has to raise the load slightly at full arm's extension to get it over the conveyor's edge. Most of the work is done by the weaker muscles of grip and the shoulders.

In many situations it is not possible to push or pull the load directly in front of the body. Instead it is moved across the front of the body using a lateral push. The amount of strength available for pushing an object across the body is very small, limited primarily to the weaker shoulder muscles (pectoralis, especially). Forces exceeding 15 lbs (67 Newtons) in this direction are difficult for many people to exert. This value is not the weight of the object to be moved but, rather, is the force to slide it across the work surface. Anything that can reduce the frictional resistance of the object and the surface should make the task more acceptable.

In a seated workplace it is often necessary to move a tray, a part, or the product from one side of the workplace to the other. It is generally recommended that objects weighing more than 10 lbs (4.5 kg) should be handled while standing. To improve handling efficiency, these workplaces are often designed to permit the worker to slide the object or tray on and off of a conveyor at the rear of the workplace. This sliding force should be kept below 30 lbs (134 Newtons).

In the design of tasks where force exertion is used to slide objects rather than having to lift them, it is important to avoid workspace confinement (such as inadequate foot room) that might result in twisting. Lateral motions are more likely to unevenly load the spine and result in twisting than are straight-forward motions. Forward pushes from a seated workplace may put some additional strain on the back if the worker leans forward in his or her chair and cannot use a footrest effectively (Figure III-17c). Low sliding resistance and whole body forward pushes are preferable.

Section III: How the Workplace Can Be Improved

CHAPTER 8: SPECIAL WORKPLACE AIDS FOR PEOPLE WITH LOW BACK PAIN

Some of the work activities and workplace design factors that may bring out back pain symptoms in people with degenerative disc disease have been reviewed in Chapter 2. Some equipment and workplace design accommodations to reduce these problems are reviewed in this chapter. They are classified under either workplace postures or manual materials handling aids.

A. WORKPLACE POSTURES

There are workplace aids that can help relieve excessive pressures on the lumbar discs by reducing the amount of bending forward, hyperextension, extended reach, or twisting. There are also ways of obtaining postural relief when doing a job that requires constant standing or sitting all day.

1. To Reduce Forward Bending and Extended Reaches

Workplace height adjustments can reduce the need for a person to bend forward over a work surface that is too low. The adjustments can be made with an adjustable table, such as a drafting table, or by using wooden platforms on the work surface to raise the work. If the latter approach is used, the platforms should be easy to remove if the next worker at the work surface prefers the fixed work height.

Extended reaches can be reduced by using tool or control extenders or aids to move objects closer. Examples of these are adapters for power tools that increase the distance from the

109

"chuck" of the driver to the screw driver bit or socket wrench. This makes it easier for an assembler or repair operator to reach points that would require awkward and extended reaches were a standard tool used. Valves or other controls may also be difficult to access in some fluid control systems, so handle extenders have also been used on them. The handle is placed at the end of a shaft that is welded to the stem of the valve (Figure III-18a). Another type of reach extender is like a shepherd's crook but with less bend in its neck. It can be fabricated from pipe and helps the worker slide an object closer to the body without having to reach far forward (Figure III-18b). Use of such an aid requires that the object can slide on its storage surface.

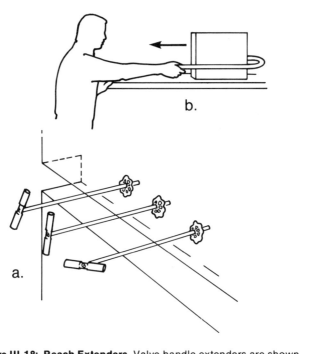

Figure III-18: Reach Extenders. Valve handle extenders are shown in "a". These are welded onto the valve stem and permit the worker to open the valve without leaning over and fully extending the arm. Use of a "crook" is shown in "b". A piece of pipe or a light, rigid, tubular material is bent to permit a case to be slid forward before it is picked up.

Special Workplace Aids for People with Low Back Pain 111

Bending forward will also occur if a person is working at too low a height. Aids that will raise the work height, such as an adjustable overhead conveyor mechanism for the part, or stools or dollies that the worker can sit on during the low work will give relief to the person with low back pain. Use of the stool or dolly depends on having leg clearance. They should not be used if hyperextension of the back or leg interference will result in more awkward postures.

2. To Reduce Hyperextension of the Back

Back hyperextension is most commonly seen when a person is working at high locations, as in overhead work, or when a bulky load is being handled. The latter category will be discussed under "Manual Materials Handling Aids" below. The primary way to reduce back hyperextension caused by too-high work levels is to raise the worker above the floor using either a platform, a step stool, or a vehicle such as a platform truck (Figure III-19). Some hyperextension is inevitable in overhead work where clearances limit how much the worker can be raised. So, regular breaks from these tasks to ones that do not require hyperextension are recommended.

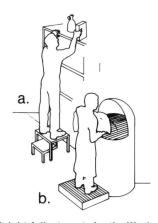

Figure III-19: Height Adjustments for the Worker. A step stool ("a") and a low platform ("b") are shown as portable aids to alter working heights and reduce stress on the back from hyperextension in too-high work.

3. To Reduce Twisting

A job that requires frequent twisting movements, even without objects being handled, is likely to bring out low back pain symptoms in people with degenerative disc disease. The reasons behind this are discussed in Chapter 3. A workplace that requires an operator to make 180-degree turns to pick up parts or product and then dispose of them is more likely to encourage trunk twisting than is one where supplies are stored adjacent to the primary work area. For assembly tasks, then, provision of storage bins or holders within a comfortable arm reach (15-20 in. or 38-51 cm) for a seated or standing operator is an approach to reduce twisting. If this is not feasible because of the nature of the task, it is important to orient the workplace so materials are as close to the main work surface as is possible. Use of roller conveyor sections to transfer parts from one area to another, especially if the parts are heavy (more than 40 pounds or 18 kgm), can also reduce the potential stress of twisting on the back (Figure III-20).

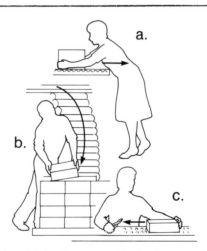

Figure III-20: Use of Roller Bearing and Roller Conveyor Sections to Reduce Handling Effort. Three examples are shown of the use of roller bearing ("a" and "c") or conveyor sections ("b") to reduce the work of transferring a product or case in the workplace. Although the worker in "b" is twisted, which is not recommended, his lower back is not experiencing as high loads because the weight of the case is carried by the conveyor.

Special Workplace Aids for People with Low Back Pain

Use of a swivel chair in a seated workplace will reduce the opportunities for trunk twisting when parts are procured or disposed of. This assumes that the feet are free to move with the chair as it swivels and are not tied to a foot pedal or restricted because of a barrier below the work surface.

4. To Provide Postural Relief in Constant Sitting or Constant Standing Jobs

Postural flexibility is a useful technique for reducing the potential for low back pain when standing or sitting is required during most of the shift. It is recommended that some seating be provided for people who mostly stand (see Figure III-22 later), and that brief standing tasks be provided for people who generally sit. In addition, the seated worker should have a footrest and good lumbar support in the chair (Figure III-21a). Footrests have been discussed in Chapter 6 as has lumbar support as a design feature of chairs. If the chair being used in the workplace does not have good lumbar support, there are a number of products available that can be placed in chairs or worn by the worker with back pain to provide that support. They include inflatable cushions that conform to the buttocks and back as one sits in a chair, rectangular foam cushions sculpted to fit the curve of the lower back (Figure III-21b), and an inflatable vest that provides a cushion for the back when one sits in a high-backed chair (Figure III-21c). Plastic supports that can be inserted in chairs and are not compressible have also been developed. The purpose of all of these aids is to support the lumbar spine and provide an alternative to a less-than-optimal chair design. Although these aids are a compromise for a well-designed chair or seat, they are portable and do offer some relief for workers with back pain who have to sit for extended periods.

For people who have to stand for the majority of the shift and do not alternate their standing with regular walking activities, a foot rail is recommended for postural relief (Figure III-22). The constant load of standing often includes some leaning forward to work on a bench, conveyor, or piece of equipment. Additional compressive force is then placed on the lumbar discs and can result in symptoms especially for people with a history of back pain. The footrail allows the worker to tilt the pelvis back and up,

Working With Backache

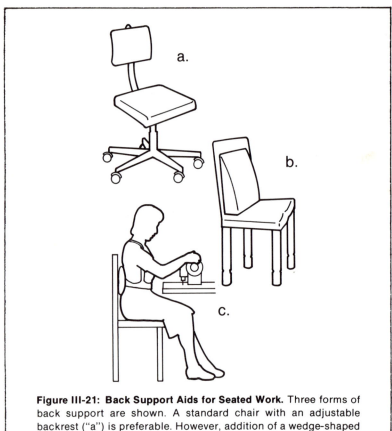

Figure III-21: Back Support Aids for Seated Work. Three forms of back support are shown. A standard chair with an adjustable backrest ("a") is preferable. However, addition of a wedge-shaped pillow ("b") to the existing chair or use of an inflatable vest that provides back support in a chair that lacks good support ("c") are ways for the back pain sufferers to overcome poor seating.

taking some of the pressure off the lumbar discs. An appropriate footrail for a standing workplace should be not more than 8 inches (20 cm) above the floor and should run the width of the work station. It should have a flat or curved surface that is at least 4 inches (10 cm) wide. If a box or portable foot support is used, it should follow the dimensions given in Chapter 6 for footrests.

B. MANUAL MATERIALS HANDLING AIDS

The lifting, holding, and carrying of objects can put high

Special Workplace Aids for People with Low Back Pain

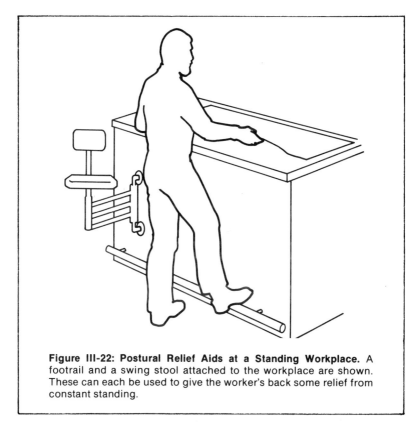

Figure III-22: Postural Relief Aids at a Standing Workplace. A footrail and a swing stool attached to the workplace are shown. These can each be used to give the worker's back some relief from constant standing.

compressive and shear forces on the lumbar discs. This may increase the reporting of low back pain, especially in people with a history of degenerative disc disease. Techniques to reduce those forces by changing the way objects are handled or moved and by reducing awkward lifts are discussed below.

1. Improving Body Postures During Handling Tasks

Bulky objects are usually handled in the workplace on an infrequent basis. These may be large in several dimensions, such as a roll of insulation material, or may be sheet materials where it is difficult to reach across two of the dimensions. In handling such objects, the worker often hyperextends the back to reduce the stress on his or her hand, arm and shoulder muscles. One approach to reduce this hyperextension is to provide straps or special holders that permit the worker to support the load closer to the body and with a power grip. A sheet material handling aid uses a triangular holder with a D-type handle and two hooks about 18 inches (46 cm) apart that fit under the sheet. The handler carries the sheet using one hand to steady it and the other to pull up on the D-type handle with a power grip (Figure III-23).

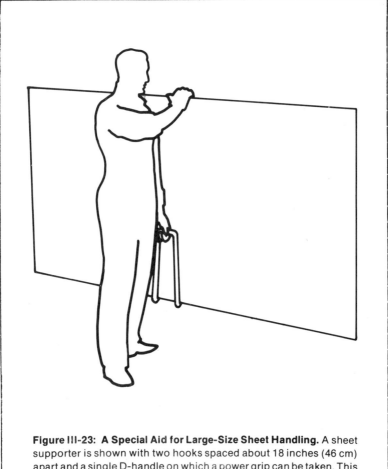

Figure III-23: A Special Aid for Large-Size Sheet Handling. A sheet supporter is shown with two hooks spaced about 18 inches (46 cm) apart and a single D-handle on which a power grip can be taken. This eliminates the need for extended reaches and pinch grip handling of the sheets and reduces the opportunities for fatigue of the forearm and shoulder muscles during sheet carrying.

Special Workplace Aids for People with Low Back Pain

If an object has to be transported for more than a few seconds a hand cart or truck is preferred, especially if the item is bulky. A sheet material cart with swivel wheels and handles at each end can be used on floors to transport several sheets at a time, for instance. Carts with one, two, or three shelves are often useful for transporting smaller items between workplaces. Wheels or dollies that are strapped to larger items such as trunks, suitcases, or business equipment reduce the need for holding and carrying materials and, thus, spare the back, arm, hand, and shoulder muscles (Figure III-24a).

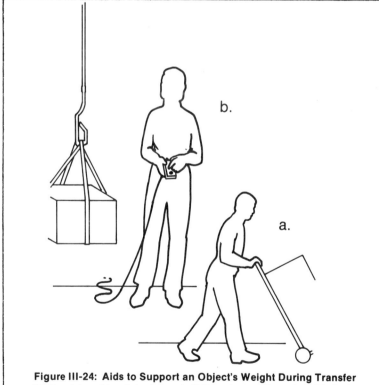

Figure III-24: Aids to Support an Object's Weight During Transfer Tasks. A hand truck is shown in "a", and a small overhead hoist is depicted in "b." Both of these aids reduce the load on the muscles by supporting the weight of the object while it is transferred from one location to another. They are recommended especially for the handling of bulky and/or heavy items or when the transfer distance is more than a few feet.

2. Reducing the Amount of Work in Handling Objects

Objects that are heavy (more than 40 lbs. or 18 kg) and have to be moved in a workplace can be a problem for people with degenerative disc disease. Handling aids such as hoists may be useful in supporting the object during transfer so the worker only has to direct the load, not lift and hold it (Figure III-24b). If a hoist is not available, equipment that will raise the load so it can be transferred at about waist level to the next location is recommended: examples are levelators, lowerators, and scissors lifts. The levelators and scissors lifts have powered adjustment capability and can be moved by each worker to the best height for handling (Figure III-25). They are often placed under pallets or skids and the levels are changed as the product is put on or taken off. The lowerator is spring-loaded, and the weight of objects placed on it pushes the spring down, keeping the loading level constant. Storage carts for plates in many cafeterias use this principle. Low lifts are avoided and less bending forward is needed when a levelator, scissors table, or lowerator is available.

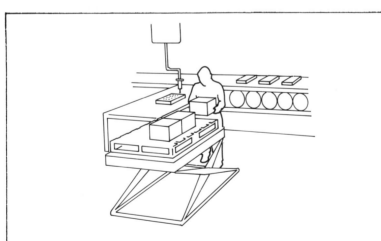

Figure III-25: A Load Levelling Aid for Manual Handling Tasks. A scissors lift table is illustrated (the guard at its base has been removed to illustrate the scissors mechanism) as it is being used in a final aseembly work station. The product is assembled, packed into a case and transferred horizontally to the pallet on the scissor lift. As the pallet is loaded, the lift table is lowered to that horizontal transfers are possible throughout the handling activity.

Special Workplace Aids for People with Low Back Pain 119

When highly repetitive lifting is required, adjustable height aids like levelators are also recommended because they reduce the total workload. Each time an item is lifted from a low height, as when pallets are unloaded near floor level, the body is also lifted. The work of raising the body makes up a substantial part of the job workload, and this effort is not contributing to productivity. In repetitive lifting tasks it is also recommended that ways be found to slide the object rather than lifting it. The use of a section of roller conveyor to transfer a part or product from one part of the workplace to another has already been mentioned. An air table or a roller bearing table surface can also be used to aid in sliding an item so it does not have to be lifted. These are particularly helpful for workplaces where bulky loads are moved. The air table contains compressed air in small metal jets that are mounted in the work surface. The sheet materials or cases move over the surface with little frictional resistance and can be directed to the next location. Roller bearing tables are particularly useful for case or carton handling tasks as they reduce the frictional resistance for sliding. Highly polished (waxed) maple surfaces and the additional of "slides" made of Teflon or other materials have also been used to aid in sliding items across work surfaces so that lifting is not required.

Where it is difficult to justify the purchase of a levelator or scissors table, use of additional pallets or of a fixed platform is recommended to raise the height of a supply or outgoing pallet-load of parts. Placing 2 pallets under the pallet being unloaded will raise the lower tier to at least 16 inches above the floor instead of having it 5-6 inches above the floor during lifting. This reduces compressive force on the lumbar discs during lifting and reduces leg interference during the initial procurement of the item. If the parts arrive in a large bin (more than 30 inches (76 cm) to a side), use of a fixture that can tilt the bin forward about 45 degrees reduces the horizontal location of the lifts at the far side of the bin and the extended reaches to the bin's bottom.

The choice of aids or workplace modifications to reduce stress on the back for persons with low back pain will depend on the frequency of handling, duration of the tasks, and the weight and dimensions of the objects handled. The above techniques are examples of an approach intended to reduce the compressive and shear forces on the lower spine and to prevent fatigue of the trunk muscles that support it. Self-paced, well-designed lifting tasks are not out of the question for a person with degenerative disc disease.

Section IV: How the Job Can Be Improved

Chapter 9: The Size and Design of Objects to Be Handled

Chapter 10: Providing Adequate Recovery Time

Chapter 11: Work Patterns and Job Design

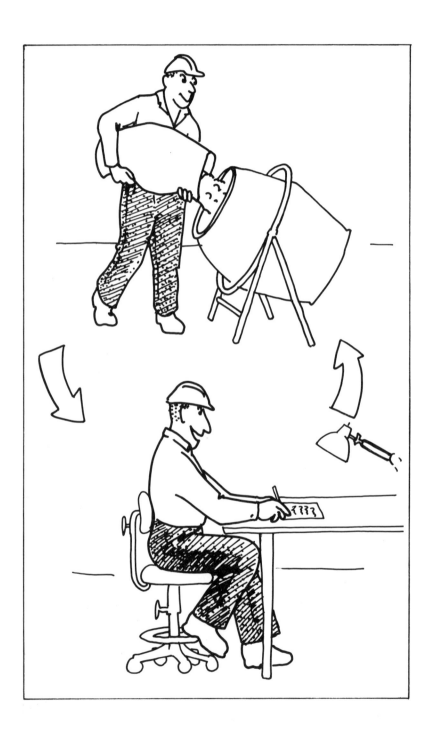

Section IV: How the Job Can Be Improved

In addition to activities by the workers and workplace modifications, administrative and job design approaches can be used to improve the work situation for a person with low back pain. These approaches are widely appropriate because they reduce the opportunities for muscle fatigue to develop. Included in this section is a discussion of the design of items to be handled, including load size, configuration, and handhold characteristics. The rest of the section addresses job design, providing adequate recovery time in more demanding physical or postural work, and structuring the job to allow a person with low back pain to regulate the work pattern in accordance with his or her capacity for physical effort.

CHAPTER 9: THE SIZE AND DESIGN OF OBJECTS TO BE HANDLED

The size of an object that has to be lifted or carried and whether it has good handholds will determine the amount of stress on the lower back. Bulky objects are more difficult to handle and often result in strong hyperextension of the back. The handler arches back to bring the load closer to the center of the body so as to enhance the postural stability. As a result, the compressive forces on the posterior third of the L5 (fifth lumbar) disc are increased, and there is an increased risk of damage to the disc. If an object does not have handholds, the handler has to find the most stable location to grip it. The strength available for gripping will depend on the dimensions over which the grip is taken and on other characteristics of the surface and object size. If a grip is not stable or fatigues quickly, there is a risk of losing control of the load and having to either shift it to other muscles or drop it. These shifts or drops may be accompanied by awkward postures, uneven loading of the spine, or sudden, unguarded movements that may aggravate back pain symptoms in people with degenerative disc disease. In this chapter some suggestions for object size and handhold design are included both for packaging and container designers to use in developing their designs and for back pain sufferers to use in determining when they should look for alternate ways of handling the object.

A. DIMENSIONS OF THE LOAD

The dimensions of an object that has to be manually handled will determine which muscle groups are most heavily stressed and what posture is assumed. Objects that are compact, i.e., less than 10 inches (25 cm) to a side, can be held close to the body without requiring the elbows to be abducted (held away from the sides) and without overloading the shoulder muscles. When the length of an object exceeds 18 inches (46 cm), the handler's elbows will be abducted and the shoulders will be loaded, because 18 inches is wider than the usual shoulder breadth. If the object is handled across its length, the elbows cannot be kept flat against the body and must be elevated (Figure IV-1).

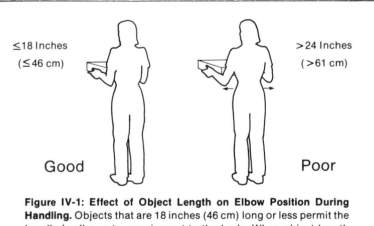

Figure IV-1: Effect of Object Length on Elbow Position During Handling. Objects that are 18 inches (46 cm) long or less permit the handler's elbows to remain next to the body. When object length exceeds 18 inches, and especially at values above 24 inches (61 cm), the elbows are abducted and the shoulder muscles can fatigue and limit handling times.

The Size and Design of Objects to be Handled 125

As the widths of objects increase from 10 to 20 inches (25-51 cm), the location of the load's center of mass is moved forward, and this puts more stress on the lower back (Figure IV-2). The biomechanics of this have been presented in Chapter 5. In addition, the wider the load, the more it has to be supported by shoulder muscles and the less effective are the stronger upper arm muscles (biceps and triceps). At an object width of 36 inches when the weight has to be supported 18 inches (46 cm) or more in front of the body, shoulder strength is the primary limiter of the weight that can be safely lifted. In general, it is recommended that object width be kept near 10 inches (25 cm) when there is a choice.

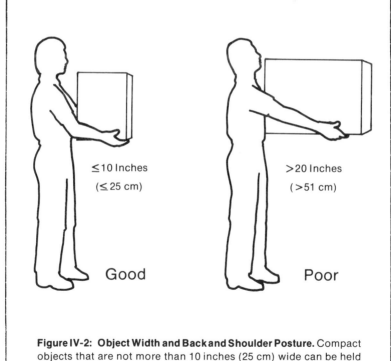

≤10 Inches
(≤25 cm)

Good

>20 Inches
(>51 cm)

Poor

Figure IV-2: Object Width and Back and Shoulder Posture. Compact objects that are not more than 10 inches (25 cm) wide can be held close to the body and do not put an additional postural load on the back and shoulders. Objects that are wider than this, especially at widths of more than 20 inches (51 cm), put heavy forces on the lumbar discs and often cause hyperextension of the worker's back during handling.

The depth of an object will determine where it is carried and how stable it is as it is lifted. If it does not have good handholds and has to be lifted from the bottom, the depth of the object will strongly influence the height of the hands and the posture of the trunk during the lift. If the object has to be carried, its depth may interfere with walking and will require the carrier to hold it out farther in front of the body. This increases the pressure on the lumbar discs and cannot be sustained for very long. A depth of about 6 inches (15 cm) is optimal to avoid interference with walking and to provide stability. Since many parts and products are deeper than this, a guideline of 12 inches (30 cm) in depth or less for the design of packages may be more practical. If handholds are provided, the depth may be greater and still provide stable handling, but then interference with the legs must be evaluated in relation to handhold positions.

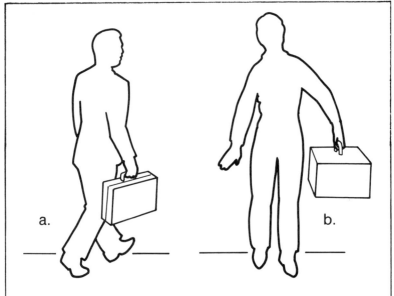

Figure IV-3: Object Depth and One-Handed Carrying Postures. The arm, shoulder, and trunk postures are shown for a person carrying a compact (less than 4 inches or 10 cm deep) briefcase ("a") and for a person carrying an item with a handhold at the top that is both wide and deep ("b"). The bulky item causes shoulder fatigue and unequal loading of the spine; this can result in low back pain for people with recurrent symptoms.

The Size and Design of Objects to be Handled 127

If the object is carried in one hand, e.g., a suitcase, its width or depth is even more important. The deeper it is, the greater is the load on the shoulder muscles to keep it away from the legs during walking (Figure IV-3). The handler also leans to the opposite side in order to reduce arm stress, and this motion unevenly loads the spine. The shoulder work results in rapid fatigue of these muscles. If the object's width is 4 inches (10 cm) or less, the arm can support the load without shoulder abduction being required.

B. CONFIGURATION OF THE LOAD

If the object to be moved is within the size guidelines given above, it still may be difficult to handle because of its configuration. If its weight is not distributed equally but is concentrated on one side (Figure IV-4a), the handler has to adjust posture to balance the load during its transfer. In some situations the balancing may be done by unequally loading the trunk, thereby reducing the stability of the spine. A person with a history of low back pain will usually avoid unequal weighting of the spine as would occur if a heavy suitcase is carried in one hand and nothing is held to counteract it in the other hand. Handling a piece of equipment with a motor in one end, for instance, may put shear forces on the lower discs that could aggravate back pain symptoms in these workers.

If the object to be lifted contains liquid or powder that can shift as it is moved, additional stress is placed on the back, hand, arm, and shoulder muscles (Figure IV-4b). The unstable load may result in compensatory movements of the trunk to counteract a sudden shift in the load. These unguarded movements can be associated with increased risk of low back pain.

Because poorly configured objects may still have to be handled, there are some techniques that can be used to reduce the effects mentioned above. Powders, grains, and pellets or other chemicals that can shift when handled should be placed in bags that match their volume, wherever possible, so weight shifting is less severe. Some of these substances are handled in bulk containers such as fiber drums and large boxes; these do not need to be lifted but can be rolled ("chimed") or transported by a forklift or pallet truck to their destinations. Objects with unequal weight distribution that may not be apparent when one looks at them should be marked to indicate the heavier side. Suggested handling locations can also be marked if the items do not have built-in handholds.

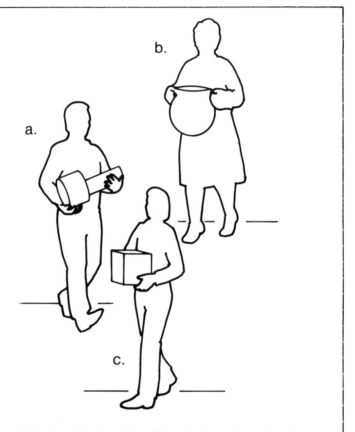

Figure IV-4: Load Configurations. Three loads are shown. An object with uneven weight distribution is shown in "a", a woman carrying a kettle of liquid is shown in "b", and a person carrying a compact load is shown in "c". The uneven load puts additional stress on the back and abdominal muscles to stabilize the spine. The shifting liquid has to be held out from the body. It can cause a sudden shift of the center of mass of the upper body and the load that the back or abdominal muscles will have to counteract.

Section IV: How the Job Can Be Improved

CHAPTER 10: PROVIDING ADEQUATE RECOVERY TIME

Earlier chapters have discussed the relationship between the intensity of muscle work and the time it can be sustained before some recovery time must be provided. More intense, or harder, muscle work results in some build-up of lactic acid and temporary depletion of the muscle energy supplies. These have to be "paid back" between muscle efforts. Thus, the distribution of lighter effort tasks within a job that includes heavy effort tasks can influence the build-up of fatigue and the ability of the worker to continue the work for a full shift. In this chapter, the implications of fatigue in the muscles that stabilize the spine and the need for postural relief and proper design of manual handling tasks is discussed.

A. MUSCLE FATIGUE AND SPINAL STABILITY

The importance of fitness of the back was described in Chapter 3. The more fit these muscles are, the higher their strength capacity, and the lower the percentage of strength a given task will take. Lower %MVC (maximum voluntary contraction of muscle) activities can be sustained for longer times before fatigue occurs (see Figure II-11 in Chapter 3).

As a muscle fatigues, the same amount of load will become a greater part of its capacity. This continues until the load and the capacity are identical and the effort can only be sustained for a few seconds more. Good job design tries to reduce the probability that muscles will fatigue to this point by giving the most heavily loaded muscles in a task some relaxation time in order to restore their energy supplies. Intermittent work is the alternation of heavy and light work (or rest) in such a way as to limit the build-up of lactic acid over time.

The muscles that support and align the lower spine are active in maintaining upright posture and in performing manual handling tasks. An awkward posture, such as bending forward to work on a too-low surface or leaning to one side to make an extended reach with one hand, will require work of the back, hip, and abdominal muscles. The longer the posture has to be maintained, the more chance there is for these muscle groups to fatigue. When they are fatigued, they are less able to stabilize the spine in a subsequent task, e.g., in handling product or exerting forces on one side of the body. To assess the stress on the back in a job, therefore, one has to look at not only the required lifts and postures but also at the length of time when a non-optimal posture is taken before making a lift or taking a more extreme posture. This possible fatigue of the important spine stabilizers during a job may help to explain why some jobs with only moderately heavy handling tasks show higher low back pain incidence reporting than jobs with heavier loads.

If the erector spinae and hip extensor muscles are fatigued from constant bending, a twist of the trunk or high compressive forces on the lower lumbar discs produced by a heavy lift may result in misalignment of the spine. The person with degenerative disc disease who already has some instability in his or her lower spine due to fluid loss from the L4 or L5 disc will be particularly vulnerable to fatigue of these muscles. The misalignment may trap the nerve root between the vertebral processes and cause irritation and pain. Irritation of the nerve root may set up a reflex increase in the strength of contraction of the back muscles and can create a muscle spasm that is very painful. To relieve the spasm, the person has to stretch out the muscle right away by curling the trunk forward and trying to mechanically realign the vertebrae to take the pressure off of the nerve root. Ice packs and, later, hot packs are sometimes used to temporarily relieve the spasm. The less fit the back muscles are, or the more fatigued they are from an awkward posture or inadequate recovery time between exertions, the greater the opportunity for improper alignment of the spine and a subsequent nerve root pinch.

B. POSTURAL RELIEF

Extended periods of work in one posture can result in static muscle fatigue even when heavy work is not required. The muscle loading would have to be less than 15% of maximum strength to avoid fatigue after 5 minutes of continuous work (see Chapter 3, Figure II-11). Even in jobs where one's posture is relatively restricted, as in long-distance truck driving, there is a natural adjustment of posture every few minutes. This movement relieves the static load from some muscles and brings in other muscles to do the task.

The importance of chair and seat design to allow a person to adjust posture laterally as well as vertically and horizontally has been discussed in Chapter 6. Provision of an adjustable backrest that will move in as the worker leans forward on the work surface, for instance, is a recommended chair design feature for jobs requiring continuous sitting. Footrest availability, especially a portable design, is also recommended as it gives the worker more options for height adjustment in the workplace. For a continuous standing job, provision of a footrail or a support stool has been recommended to offer some relief for the leg, buttock, and back muscles.

If options for changing posture are provided, most people will not require additional recovery time in constant standing or constant sitting jobs. When awkward postures such as leaning to one side, bending forward, squatting, crouching, or twisting the trunk are required, however, additional recovery time is needed to prevent loss of strength in the trunk and buttock muscles over time. Figure IV-5 illustrates the recovery time needed (vertical axis) after muscle exertions of different intensities (curves) for several durations (horizontal axis) of continuous work. A person working in a bent-over posture that loads the erector spinae muscles to 40% of their maximum capacity, therefore, will need more recovery time the longer he or she remains in that posture (i.e., 5 minutes of recovery time after 1 minute of bending) in order to avoid fatigue of those muscles. Bending for more than 1 minute at a time at this work intensity will fatigue the muscles and may require up to 45 minutes of recovery time if the muscles are exhausted.

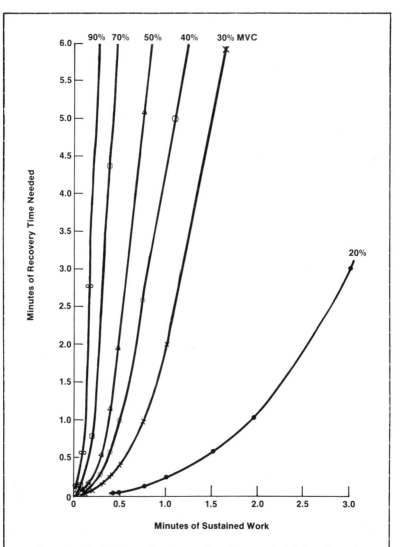

Figure IV-5: Recovery Times as a Function of Work Intensity and Duration. The amount of recovery time, in minutes on the vertical axis, that is needed to recover from a muscle effort of a given duration, in minutes on the horizontal axis, is shown for different muscle work intensitites (% of maximum voluntary contraction strength) by a series of curves. Use of these curves is illustrated in the text later in this chapter. Light muscle effort is represented by the 20% and 30% curves, moderate effort by the 40% and 50% curves, and heavy effort by the 70% and 90% curves.

Providing Adequate Recovery Time

In methods analyses of job demands it has been common to award a 10-15% fatigue factor for people who are required to work in awkward postures. This provides about one hour of recovery time per shift and should be adequate in a self-paced job where the work and recovery pattern can be regulated by the worker. It is probably a less satisfactory approach in externally-paced operations. There the worker has less control over work and recovery patterns and may get the fatigue factor time allowance in 10-15 minute blocks at the end of about an hour of continuous work in the awkward posture. Short work periods broken up by short recovery periods or by work that uses the muscles less heavily are preferable to intensive, long-duration work and long recovery breaks as a way of reducing the opportunity for muscles to fatigue over the shift.

C. MANUAL HANDLING TASKS AND RECOVERY NEEDS

When determining adequate recovery times for a manual handling task, one has to identify the frequency of lifting or applying force, the intensity of the work either in terms of the weight lifted or the force exerted, and the maximum duration of continuous work before a recovery break is needed. Chapter 7 includes a discussion of the interactions of these factors in the design of handling tasks. When determining how much recovery time is needed and how the work should be structured to avoid accumulating fatigue in the active muscles, one has to consider both local muscle and whole body fatigue potentials of the job. The former can be estimated from a calculation of the intensity and duration of effort of the involved muscle groups. The potential for fatigue will be related to the time of exertion and the percent of maximum muscle strength used in the postures. If the work is quite dynamic but the lifting or force exertions exceed 6 per minute, local muscle fatigue can occur unless the recovery times are adequate for moderately heavy work. Even if the static work curve (Figure II-11) suggests that the task is appropriate, the short continous muscle contraction times followed by short recovery times can still result in the build-up of some fatigue products in the muscles.

Whole body fatigue can become the limiting factor in

repetitive lifting tasks, and it is associated with demands on the heart and blood vessels (the cardiovascular system). To deliver enough oxygen to the muscles to allow them to form the energy compounds needed for muscle work, the heart rate is increased and the heart muscle has to work harder. The acceptability of working at elevated heart rates is related to the percent of maximum aerobic work capacity a person must use and the duration of the work. Figure III-15 in Chapter 7 illustrates the relationship between the percent of aerobic capacity used and time. The aerobic capacity value is specific to the type of work being done. If the work uses the whole body, as would be true in a repetitive lifting job that is done from floor to waist level, then whole body aerobic capacity as measured on a treadmill can be used to determine the individual's maximum aerobic capacity for the work. If the job involves standing quite stationary and using primarily arm, shoulder, and upper trunk muscles, then an arm capacity test, such as lifting or cranking, would be needed to assess the person's maximum aerobic capacity.

To determine the appropriate recovery periods for repetitive lifting tasks that may result in whole body fatigue, it is necessary to measure the heart rates of people during work. Enough light activities or recovery can be inserted to assure that the heart rate elevation averages no more than 33% of heart rate range (predicted maximum heart rate minus resting heart rate) for an 8-hour shift. Predicted maximum heart rates are determined by subtracting age from 220 beats per minute. With this admittedly rough estimate of aerobic work intensity, one can also look at peak work loads and be sure that they meet the guidelines for duration that Figure III-15 recommends. To bring the over-all job demands down, light activities or recovery time must be made available during the repetitive handling tasks. If oxygen usage is measured, a maximum workload of 12 ml of oxygen per minute per kilogram of body weight averaged over the 8-hour shift is recommended.

These recommendations for provision of adequate recovery time relate to low back pain in the workplace in several ways. If the posture during work is such that the back muscles are loaded not only by the weight of the object being lifted but also by the way it has to be handled, their rate of fatigue will be greater. Then

Providing Adequate Recovery Time

they may not be able to keep the spine aligned during a postural change or a sudden movement because they may not have the strength needed. As a result, there is more potential for the vertebrae to slide on one another and to pinch the nerve root during a lift or postural change, producing low back pain symptoms. If the work is very demanding and whole body fatigue occurs, the worker may be less attentive to postural changes and may slip or put an excessive load on one part of the spine. Whole body fatigue will show up as reduced endurance for work, and the worker will need longer recovery times as the shift progresses. It is better to incorporate the recovery periods into the work periods and reduce the over-all load throughout the shift than to try to make up for the heavy work with extended break times.

D. EXAMPLES OF RECOVERY TIME CALCULATIONS

Two examples of ways to calculate recovery time needs for static work and for dynamic handling tasks are given below.

1. Static Muscle Loading

If a person is doing a task that requires bending forward while working on a bench, the back muscles are likely to be loaded to about 40-50% of their capacity in order to keep the upper body from falling forward. Taking the 50% MVC value, one can find from figure II-11 that this effort can be sustained for one minute continuously. The muscle is then fatigued. If the task takes 15 seconds to complete in the bending posture, there will be slight back muscle fatigue. A recovery time of an additional 15 seconds should restore the energy supplies of the back muscles. If the static muscle load is greater, for example, 75% of maximum force, the recovery time will have to be lengthened in proportion to the work time. Fifteen seconds of bending work at 75% of the maximum strength of the back extensors will need 150 seconds of recovery time. Figure IV-5 illustrates the relationship between workload intensity, duration, and the needed recovery period to prevent accumulating fatigue. To find the proportionate recovery time after a static effort, one finds the intersection between the intensity of that effort (percent of maximum voluntary muscle strength) and the duration (or holding time in minutes). The vertical axis value at this point indicates the percent recovery time needed to restore the muscles.

2. Dynamic Work - Repetitive Manual Lifting

There are both local muscle and whole body fatigue reasons to provide adequate recovery time in these tasks. So, the first consideration is to identify the intensity and duration of the lifts and to determine the necessary recovery time using Figure IV-5, as discussed above. If the lifts are more than 6 times per minute and the object being lifted weighs more than 20 lbs (9 kg), one can calculate the additional need for recovery time by determining what the appropriate work/recovery cycle should be. For example, a 40 lb (18 kg) case may represent 75% of strength for less strong workers. The lift may only take 3 seconds, so at a steady 6 per minute lift rate, every 3 seconds of lifting is followed by 7 seconds of recovery, giving a work/recovery ratio of 1:2.5. The suggested recovery time for this task would be about 8 seconds, one more than is available at this lifting rate. An additional one second of recovery time per lift would be recommended to prevent accumulated muscle fatigue. At higher lifting frequencies additional recovery time at the end of the task would have to be given to make up for the inadequate recovery time between lifts.

To keep the total workload within acceptable levels, it is also necessary to estimate the cardiovascular load of the work. As a general guideline, one can assume a heart rate range of 100 (between resting and predicted maximum values). A heart rate elevation of 33 beats per minute above resting levels averaged over the shift is the maximum recommended workload. The heavier the handling task (more weight, higher frequency), the more light work recovery time is needed in order to reduce the total load. From a list of the energy expenditure and heart rate elevations of job activities (Table IV-1), one can determine the average and peak workloads and assure that they stay within the guidelines in Figure III-15 (Chapter 7) by adding light work as needed. For example, if a job requires a worker to lift heavy boxes at 6 per minute for 4 hours a shift, and the average heart rate elevation is 50 beats per minute, that represents a 50/100 or 50% of aerobic capacity (represented by % of heart rate range) workload. To reduce the total workload to 33% of maximum for

Providing Adequate Recovery Time

Table IV-1: Heart Rate Elevations in Several Occupational Tasks

Effort Level	Light	Moderate	Heavy	Very Heavy
HR Elevation				
Whole Body	10 - 20	21 - 45	46 - 75	>75
Upper Body	10 - 15	16 - 30	31 - 50	>50
Tasks	Typing, Data Entry (U)	Packing, Small (U)	Industrial Cleaning	Landscaping
	Record Keeping (U)	Punch Press Operation	Carpentry	Loading Coal
	Small Parts Assembly (U)	Metal Working (U)	Plastering	Handling Cases, >25 lbm > 4/min.
	Drill Press Operation (U)	Painting	Sweeping/ Mopping Floors	Cement Mixing
	Sitting, Reading	Driving a Truck/Car	Gardening	Stone Masonry
	Monitoring	Sewing (U)	Packing, Large (U)	Smelting Work
	Standing	Ironing (U)	Sheet Metal Work	Agricultural Work
	Drafting	Washing Windows	Laundry Operations (U)	
	Inspecting	Bench Work	Truck and Auto Repair	
		Sorting Scrap	Road Paving	
		Walking	Metal Casting	
		Crane Operation (U)		
		Cafeteria Work (U)		
		Machine Tending		

Table IV-1: Heart Rate Elevations In Several Occupational Tasks. Estimates of heart rate elevations (beats/min above the resting value) for work tasks are given in four effort categories from light to very heavy work. These can be used to design jobs so that the total workload does not exceed the aerobic capacity guidelines presented in Figure III-15 (Chapter 7). For upper body work (U), local muscle fatigue should also be evaluated for moderately heavy or heavier tasks.

the whole shift, the 50% would have to be balanced by a very low workload. That value can be calculated by solving the following equation:

$$(50)(240 \text{ min.}) + (x)(240) = (33)(480)$$
$$12{,}000 + 240x = 15840$$
$$240x = 3840$$
$$x = 16.0$$

A 16% of aerobic capacity workload is not much more than light assembly or paper work. This suggests that if the heavy lifting is done for the first four hours of the shift, the workers can only do light work during the second half.

This example illustrates why short duration intensive effort is preferable to long duration effort with added rest break time. If the above task were to be broken up into 10 minute segments with 5 minutes of lighter activity alternating for the full 8 hours, the lifting frequency could be reduced from 6 per minute to 4.5 per minute, the heart rate elevation would be reduced from 50 to about 38 beats per minute (a 25% drop in workload), and the light activity could be about 23% of maximum aerobic capacity in order to average out at 33% for the shift. The calculation is as follows:

$$38(320) + x(160) = 33(480)$$
$$12160 + 160x = 15840$$

$$160x = 3680$$
$$x = 23\% \quad \text{moderate activity level}$$

A number of moderately demanding jobs can be done using 23% of aerobic work capacity, including wrapping and packing tasks, some cleaning operations, moderate effort assemblies, and many inspection and monitoring tasks.

By altering the pattern of work in this example, one also reduces the stress on local muscle groups by giving more recovery time between lifts. Total output per shift is not reduced, although it is taking more of the shift to complete the work. There may be jobs where this ability to restructure the pattern of work is not possible. Those jobs will also probably require some "natural

Providing Adequate Recovery Time 141

selection" of workers because they will be too difficult for people with lower work capacity to perform. When a second worker is available, the heavier work can often be shared. Thus, more recovery time is provided by cutting the lifting frequency in half for each worker.

Section IV: How the Job Can Be Improved

CHAPTER 11: WORK PATTERNS AND JOB DESIGN

The previous chapter discussed ways of alternating light and strenuous tasks to reduce the local muscle stress and the whole body demands of repetitive tasks and awkward postures. In this chapter the implications of self-paced and externally-paced jobs for the person with low back pain are discussed. In addition, some guidelines are included for the choice of job activities and the design of jobs to reduce the opportunities for muscle or whole body fatigue.

A. WORK AND RECOVERY PATTERNS IN SELF—PACED WORK

Determination of the job effort level that is acceptable to most workers will depend on the strengths and postures required, the total energy required over the shift, the environmental stressors present, and the amount of control the worker has over the way the work is done. Physiological and psychological "behaviors" modify the way a job is done, sometimes greatly different from its initial design. For example, if a person (not a machine) is pacing a handling job, he or she may cluster the lifting into a short, intensive period and then do lighter and less strenuous tasks for longer periods between the lifting tasks. This strategy is in lieu of doing fewer lifts over a longer time period. If the person has low back pain, however, it may be more suitable to intersperse the lighter activities more frequently within the lifting periods. Figure IV-6 illustrates some of these potential work patterns. The person with backache is responding to the accumulating fatigue in the back muscles caused by the repetitive lifting; he or she is protecting the back by reducing the continuous lifting time to a level where fatigue is not significant. The person with no backache is lifting to "get it over with" and to have a longer period to do other tasks or relax before the next lifting period occurs.

Well-designed jobs will permit the work to be accomplished during the shift by any one of a number of job patterns. The appropriateness of an intensive lifting period will be determined by the nature of the materials being handled and by the fitness of the handler. Such a work pattern should not be required since many people of less strength or less endurance capacity will not be able to follow such a pattern without fatigue.

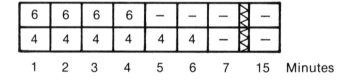

Figure IV-6: Lifting Patterns for People With and Without Low Back Pain. Examples are shown of possible self-paced lifting patterns for workers without ("a") and with ("b") low back pain on a job where frequent moderately heavy lifting is required. The theoretical job requirement is unloading 24 cases weighing 20 pounds (9 kg) each from a pallet every 15 minutes throughout the shift.

Work Patterns and Job Design

Even if a handling task is not required or is well within most people's capabilities, postural requirements may put the person with back pain at a disadvantage in some jobs. If the job is self-paced, he or she can usually find a way to get postural relief by alternating activities frequently. A repair bench worker, for instance, can work for several minutes while seated on a stool at the bench. He or she can get up and procure a new product or dispose of the old one, do paper work, or do another test in the standing posture at a higher work bench in order to get postural relief. Conversations with fellow workers, a search for a better tool, trips to the drinking fountain or restrooms, and other legitimate activities also serve as breaks from the primary task. If the job has been structured to make it unnecessary for the worker to leave his or her workbench or station, these secondary work activities and arbitrary work breaks often increase in order to provide the postural adjustments that most people need.

B. PACED WORK AND WORK PATTERNS

There are many types of paced work. Some of these are paced by the worker and include a desire to meet a particular goal, conscientiousness, and a desire to excel or "be the best." Some are paced by supervision and relate to production goals, incentive pay, deadlines, and standards of performance. Others are a function of the workplace and job characteristics, such as conveyor pacing, emergency responses, service needs, and rapid response computer systems. Work that is paced by the worker, by supervision, or by the job goals (such as rapid service) can be structured to fit the capabilities of many workers unless the time constraints are unreasonably tight. Work that is machine-paced or that requires emergency responses cannot be organized as well by the worker. The way such work is designed will determine how many people will be able to do it.

Chapter 10 includes a discussion of the importance of providing adequate recovery time in a job where moderately heavy or heavy effort tasks are done or where awkward postures are required. In an externally-paced task the recovery time is fixed; if it is not adequate, the worker has to find ways to get away from the machine in order to recover fully. Some of the arbitrary and secondary work breaks mentioned above, such as getting a drink of water, going to the restroom, or getting a new tool are used to get away from the pace pressure. Since no piece of machinery is routinely 100% efficient, occasional breakdowns in the line will also provide work breaks from the pace pressure. If the work is on a reasonably short line (6-12 people on a work team), the line may be stopped infrequently by the lead operator in order to give the worker a break while some maintenance or a new set-up is done. Occasionally a line is stopped just to allow people to "catch up."

A person with chronic low back pain is at a disadvantage in externally-paced operations because there are fewer options for organizing the work pattern to reduce back stress. If the product is moving in and out of the workplace at a fixed rate, it is harder to take frequent short breaks, to readjust posture, or to rest the muscles involved in a lifting task. Because the worker cannot control these factors as well in machine-paced operations, it is important to include a variety of activities and postures in the tasks done at each station. One should also consider the option of moving people between stations in order to spread out the heavier tasks and to make the jobs suitable for more people.

C. JOB DESIGN GUIDELINES

The guidelines for job design given below focus on two primary needs of the person with backache, providing postural relief and permitting the person to vary his or her work pattern in physically demanding jobs.

1. Do not confine a worker to one location for the full shift, but provide alternatives for moving to other places in order to get supplies, do record keeping tasks, or do quality checks, for example.

2. Provide for postural adjustments during the work. Have some type of seating available for predominantly standing activities and include some activities that require standing or walking in a job that is done at a seated workplace.

3. For self-paced jobs with frequent moderately heavy to heavy lifting tasks (see Chapter 7), provide ways to break the lifting tasks into 5- to 15-minute periods with less demanding

Work Patterns and Job Design   147

tasks alternating for equal lengths of time. Ideally, the structuring of these tasks should be loose enough to allow each person to develop his or her own best work pattern. The job designer has to define some light work activities that are integral to the job and can be used as recovery periods between the heavier tasks.

    4. For externally-paced jobs such as conveyor assembly lines, decisions about the time needed to do the task and which activities go into each job should consider the need for adequate recovery time in moderately heavy or heavy handling tasks (see Chapter 10). Line balancing should consider both the time to accomplish the task and the time needed to recover before the next task is done. Enough light activities to provide adequate recovery time should be scheduled in the heavier jobs.

    5. In machine-paced operations where materials are coming in and out of a workplace by conveyor, the worker should be able to work in places other than directly at his or her work station. It should be possible to work down the line a little in order to permit more variability in performance when parts do not fit properly or when distractions, such as visitors, are present. When a supplying activity is scheduled to occur and the worker needs to get a little ahead on the line, he or she should be able to work up the line, too.

    6. If an object weighs more than 40 lbs (18 kg), find a way to slide it rather than requiring it to be lifted. This is especially true if the handling is done more than once a minute for much of the shift.

SECTION V

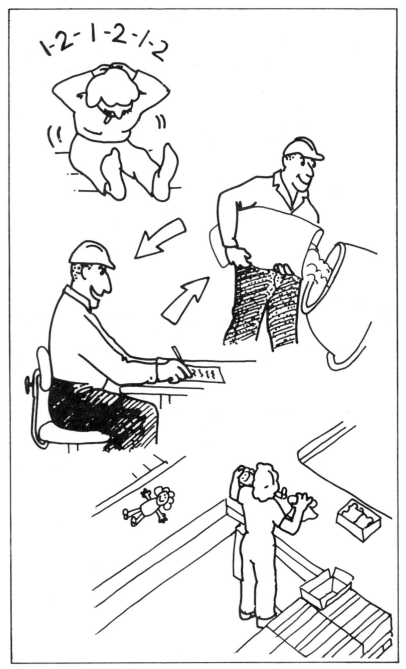

Section V: Summary and Addenda

CHAPTER 12: SUMMARY

In looking at the low back pain problem in industry, one should recognize that there are ways that the lost time and disability can be reduced through actions of the worker, the workplace and job design engineers, and supervision. The worker who has repeated low back pain episodes can learn good body mechanics, avoid actions that may trigger the attacks ("aggravators"), follow safe work practices in lifting and handling materials, and do regular exercises to keep the body muscles toned, especially those of the back, hips and abdomen. The design engineers can help the person with low back pain by assuring that reaches are within most people's capabilities without having to stretch or twist, that working heights do not result in static loading of the back, that handling requirements are resonable, and that postural flexibility is provided. Supervision can improve the low back problem in industry by supporting improvements in workplaces or jobs where static loading or twisting of the back may aggravate symptoms in people with degenerative disc disease. They can also learn to recognize job and environmental pressures that make it more necessary for a worker to report low back pain episodes. These include externally-paced operations and tight time lines, jobs where the worker has little control over the way the work is done, and situations where postural relief is difficult to obtain. In addition, managers can encourage the establishment of worker fitness programs, especially for people who work in jobs that require moderately heavy to heavy effort or awkward postures.

A. NEW DESIGN

A long-term approach to reducing low back pain disability is to design the workplace so there is less opportunity for the "aggravators" of symptoms to occur. A summary of design guidelines that should make it less necessary to report low back pain symptoms is given below.

1. Keep working heights around elbow height for most people. For standing work this is in a height range from about 35 to 41 inches (89 to 104 cm) above the floor. For seated work it is from 7 to 11 inches (18 to 28 cm) above the seat pan of the chair or stool.

2. Keep forward reaches within 15 inches (38 cm) of the front of the body and between elbow and head height, roughly from 38 to 55 inches (97 to 140 cm) above the floor when standing. Higher and lower forward reaches are not recommended, especially on a repetitive basis. If they occur, forward reaches of more than 10 inches require bending and stretching and increase the discomfort for people with low back pain.

3. Avoid lifting items above 50 inches (127 cm) or below 20 inches when standing, where possible. Use sliding for low lifts or use levelators to raise the load above 20 inches for handling tasks.

4. Design force exertion tasks so they can be approached directly in front of the body and at 40 to 50 inches (102 to 127 cm) above the floor.

5. If a compact object weighs more than 40 lb (18 kg), look for ways to handle it other than lifting. Use conveyors or sliding surfaces, for example.

6. Provide workplace aids for postural relief, such as foot supports, chairs or support stools, armrests, and backrest cushions, as appropriate to the work. Design jobs so the seated operator can get up and walk and the standing operator can sit down occasionally.

7. Design packaging so the dimensions do not exceed the

reach and grip capabilities of most people and so the package does not interfere with the legs during walking and carrying. Objects that have more than two dimensions that exceed 20 inches (57 cm), even if they weigh less than 25 lbs (11 kg), may be difficult for less strong workers to handle repetitively.

8. Orient the workplace so that twisting of the upper body is not likely to occur. Keep the work within a 90-degree movement pattern where possible. Store supplies so they can be accessed without the worker having to take awkward postures, preferably between 20 and 55 inches (51 and 140 cm) above the floor in a standing workplace. Storage at or up to 25 inches (64 cm) above the work surface in a seated workplace is also preferred. Supplies that are only occasionally needed can be placed far enough to one side to require the worker to stand up and get some postural relief.

9. Select a chair according to the type of work being done and the time of continuous sitting. The longer a person has to remain seated before he or she can get up to walk or stand for a while, the more important it is to have a chair with good back and foot support and with adjustability to improve the workplace "fit" for the individual worker.

10. Provide aids for handling materials that are not compact or are heavier than 40 lbs (18 kg). Small hoists, straps, carts, and transfer tables with roller bearings are examples of such aids.

11. Include height adjustability in standing workplace work surfaces, where feasible.

B. EXISTING WORKPLACES

Workplace problems can often be identified by looking at accident and medical reports for low back pain incidents. Jobs that involve heavy lifting, awkward postures, or high time pressure demands that make work organization difficult for the individual worker may show higher low back pain reporting than do lighter, more sedentary jobs. The need for a person to report symptoms when a low back pain episode occurs is much greater if the job activities put fairly high pressures on the lumbar discs or contribute to fatigue of the spinal musculature.

It may sometimes be difficult to alter the workplace to fit the recommended guidelines for working heights, reaches, orientation, etc. Accommodation of individuals according to their back problems may be a more feasible approach in some instances to help get a person back to work or to reduce the potential for aggravating his or her symptoms on the job. Most of these accommodations will be useful for people without back problems, too, as they reduce static loading of muscles that can limit self-paced productivity levels. Some accommodations are described below.

1. Use a scissors lift, levelator, platform, or 2 or 3 extra pallets to raise items to about 20 inches (51 cm) above the floor in frequent handling tasks.

2. Use tool or reach extenders to reduce the need to stretch or twist in long reaches.

3. Provide chair inserts or inflatable cushions for additional lumbar support at a seated workplace if the chair is not designed according to ergonomic guidelines.

4. Use an adjustable footrest, or use a block of wood, styrofoam, or a telephone book as a footrest for standing or sitting workplaces to give postural relief.

5. Use small light platforms on a too-low work surface to raise the work height enough to reduce bending for the taller worker.

6. Use sections of roller conveyor, ball bearings mounted on the work surface, or slides to permit heavy items to be moved across the work surface without having to be lifted.

7. Include lighter activities as part of the job requirements and allow the workers to structure the way the job is performed, alternating light and heavier activities according to their best work pattern.

8. Release the person on a conveyor-paced job from the pace pressure by moving materials on and off of the conveyor line to another work surface. He or she can then keep some

Summary

control and work at an appropriate rate for the back discomfort.

9. Provide hand carts or hoists to support the weight of objects that are difficult to handle either because of their weight or their configuration.

Since about two-thirds of the workforce might experience low back pain at some point in their working careers, it is wise to take the long term approach of designing or redesigning the workplace and job so most people can work without aggravating their low back. Accommodations are appropriate as short term "fixes" and do improve the job for many people. However, integrating the ergonomic principles into the whole job will have greater benefits than simply those related to low back problems. Well-designed jobs and workplaces can improve productivity by reducing fatigue from awkward postures or too-heavy work, by providing more management flexibility in placing people in jobs and covering changing production demands, and by better using the talents and capabilities of the workers.

APPENDIX A

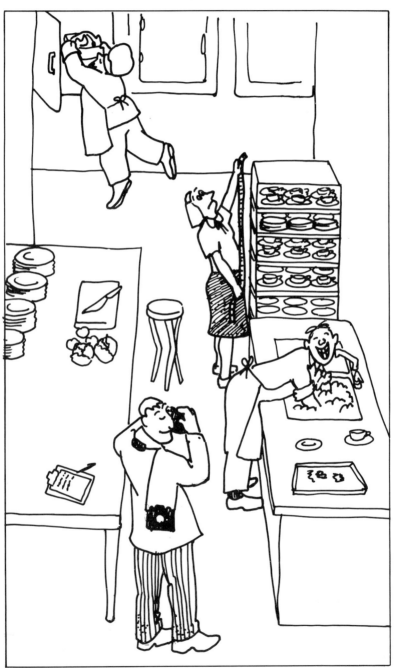

APPENDIX A: SURVEYING THE WORKPLACE

Low back pain symptoms in the workplace may not be easily prevented because of the recurrent nature of the disease. However, workplace and job situations may exacerbate symptoms by requiring the worker to use postures or handle materials that aggravate the back. This Appendix includes a checklist that can be used to help identify changes to facilitate the low back pain patient's return to the workplace. If the conditions indicated in the checklist are avoided in workplace and job design, the opportunities for extended lost time from low back pain should be reduced significantly. Other factors relating to supervisory style and conditions that may increase the risk of slip and trip accidents are also discussed.

I. Checklist to Identify Potential Low Back Pain Aggravators in the Workplace

In surveying the workplace, one should place a check by the appropriate descriptions of low back pain aggravators.

_____ 1. Constant standing with little opportunity to sit down.

_____ 2. Constant sitting with little opportunity to stand up or move around.

_____ 3. Low working heights requiring the worker to bend over frequently.

_____ 4. Extended reaches requiring the worker to bend forward to perform a task for at least a minute continuously.

Working With Backache

_____ 5. Activities that require the worker to take an awkward posture, such as crouching, while doing a task lasting longer than one minute.

_____ 6. Repeated and sustained work over shoulder level (about 50 inches above the floor).

_____ 7. Activities that require the worker to twist the upper trunk in order to reach or see something.

_____ 8. Activities that result in uneven distribution of body weight on the feet, especially where one foot is lower then the other and manual force exertion or lifting and lowering is being done.

_____ 9. Inadequate clearances for moving the feet while doing a task that will result either in uneven balance or twisting of the trunk.

_____ 10. Seating that has inadequate support for the back (no adjustable lumbar support).

_____ 11. Lack of an appropriate footrest at a seated workplace (unless working height is about 26 inches above the floor or lower).

_____ 12. A fixed workplace where it is not possible to adjust the location or heights of equipment being used, therefore possibly resulting in awkward postures for some workers (e.g., a visual display terminal that is too high or too low for some workers and cannot be tilted).

_____ 13. Occasional lifting or lowering of objects weighing more than 40 pounds at heights below 35 and above 45 inches.

_____ 14. Frequent lifting (1 per minute or more) or lowering of objects weighing more than 25 pounds.

_____ 15. Handling of large-size loads (more than 20 inches in any dimension for boxes or cases).

Appendix A-Surveying the Workplace

_____ 16. Handling of sheet materials without straps, special holders, or a second person.

_____ 17. Handling of awkward loads that can shift suddenly (such as liquids in cans or bags of loose material) when they weigh more than 25 pounds.

_____ 18. Handling of materials where the load is not shared equally between the hands, so that the load on the spine is imbalanced.

_____ 19. Sustained (more than 30 seconds) pushing or pulling of heavy loads in trucks or across flat surfaces. Forces exceeding 40 pounds (or 180 Newtons).

_____ 20. Activities that require lateral force exertion, as in pulling or pushing an object across the front of the body, where more than 15 pounds of force (70 Newtons) is required.

_____ 21. Lifting or lowering any objects when the hands are less than 10 inches above the floor, unless the knees are bent and the load is compact.

_____ 22. Externally-paced jobs where the worker cannot go "off-line" easily to take a recovery break. Examples are conveyors or production machines where the worker must keep pace or shut down the line. This is especially of concern for handling tasks.

_____ 23. Manual handling tasks that require the worker to bend to one side to exert a force or lift an object, resulting in a trunk twist or uneven loading of the spine.

_____ 24. Moderately heavy workloads that are sustained for more than 1 hour continuously, especially if a sustained awkward posture or if frequent moderately heavy to heavy lifting is required in the job.

_____ 25. Work in a cold environment (such as a food storage warehouse) where repetitive lifting or awkward postures are required.

2. Other Factors to Evaluate in the Workplace

In addition to the workplace and job factors indicated in the checklist, the work environment should be evaluated in terms of supervisory style and the potential for slip and trip accidents. The "style" factor can influence the reporting of low back pain symptoms and the ease with which a person gets back to work after an episode of low back pain. Slip and trip accidents are associated with development of or exacerbation of low back pain and may be related to either workplace or job factors.

To survey an area for its supervisory style, one has to interview the workers and supervisors and be sensitive to factors that can influence the worker's time pressure or job control. The less control or the more external pacing present, the more potential there is for a person with back problems to run into difficulties in performing the job during low back pain episodes. The difficulties arise when the person is less able to organize his or her work pattern in order to reduce back discomfort, as when he or she is constrained from taking frequent short work breaks, changing postures, using aids, or altering the methods used to accomplish the task. If a supervisor exerts close control over the way the work is done and does not tolerate work pattern adjustments, and if the person with low back pain is unable to do the work in the usual manner, then he or she will have to report the back problem and get a medical restriction. Some questions that can be used to elicit information about supervisory style are:

a. Are there any jobs in your area that might be difficult for a person with a back problem to perform?

b. How do you handle a person with a medical restriction for moderately heavy lifting (or continuous standing) in your area?

c. Are there aids available in the workplace to help in manual handling activities? Are they used?

d. Are there periods of increased production pressure when it is difficult to meet your schedule?

Appendix A-Surveying the Workplace 159

e. What is the scheduled break time on the jobs in your area? If a person completes the work early, can he or she go on break for longer periods?

An evaluation of the workplace for potential slip/trip accidents would include looking for housekeeping problems. This includes such things as: parts, liquids, or oils on the floors; crowded aisles; equipment left in walkways; and other hazards that might contribute to a tripping or slipping accident. Job factors that result in hurrying, such as too tight a timeline in a paced operation or high production pressure, are also more likely to result in slip/trip accidents. Workplaces where there is a change in the walking or standing surface height, whether it is a small flight of stairs, a stair ladder, a step stool, or a platform may also increase the risk of a slip or loss of balance because of a misstep.

This section has addressed the identification of workplace, job, and environmental factors that may contribute to low back pain problems on the job. Guidelines for designing workplaces and jobs to reduce the opportunities for aggravating backache symptoms are given in Chapters 5 through 11.

APPENDIX B

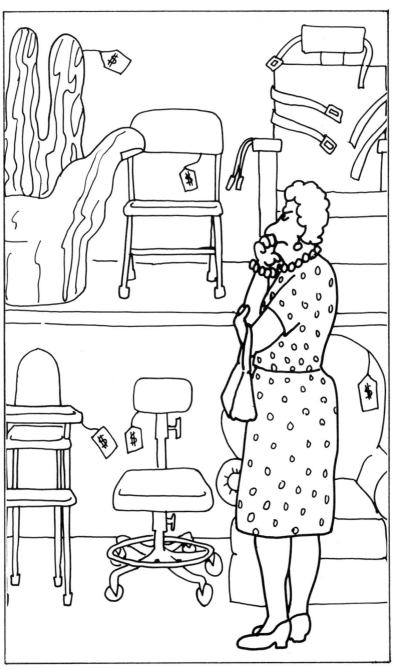

APPENDIX B: SELECTING A CHAIR

The choice of a chair for a workplace will determine how comfortable the worker is and, indirectly, how productively he or she works. This Appendix gives general guidelines for chair selection that are based on population size. It also includes information for deciding which type of chair is best as a function of the type of work being done.

1. Chair Characteristics as Selection Criteria

Table B-1 summarizes the height, width, and depth of a chair's seat, characterisitics of its back rest, and suggested dimensions for the footrest and armrests. These guidelines for selection are based on anthropometric (body size) data of the U.S. population and are intended to make it possible for the greater part of the workforce to be comfortably accommodated by the chair design. If a chair is being chosen for a personalized work station at home, the purchaser should choose one that best satisfies his or her body size.

If the height and depth recommendations for the seat are not met by available chairs, an adjustable footrest should be purchased with the chair that comes closest to the guidelines. The footrest will reduce discomfort in the back that may be caused by inadequate foot support or by an inability to use the backrest and still keep one's feet on the floor.

2. The Process of Chair Selection

The recommendations given above for selecting a chair can be used for any applications. Other decisions must be made

Working With Backache

Table B-1: Recommeded Chair and Accessory Characteristics

Characteristic	Measurement or Feature
1. Seat Height Adjustability	From 15 to 22 inches (38 to 56 cm)
2. Seat Width	17 to 19 inches (43 to 48 cm)
3. Seat Depth (or Length)	17 inches (43 cm)
4. Seat Slope	5-10 degrees up (towards the front)
5. Chair Back Rest	Lumbar and Thoracic Support
Size	6-9 inches (15-23 cm) high 12-14 inches (30-36 cm) wide
Movement Up and Down	7 to 10 inches (18-25 cm) above the seat
Movement In and Out	12 to 17 inches (30-43 cm) from the front of the seat
6. Support	5-legged; castered, if needed
7. Swivel	At least 180 degrees of swivel, if needed
8. Fabric or Chair Covering	A "breathing" fabric that does not trap heat and cause stickiness.
9. Adjustability	Easy to adjust without tools; pneumatic cylinder adjustment where possible.
10. Footrests	Portable and adjustable
Size	16 inches (41 cm) long, 12 inches (30 cm) wide
Adjustability	Easy to adjust in 2-inch (5-cm) increments
Chair Footrests	Adjustable with seat height
11. Armrests	
Size	12 inches (30 cm) long, 3 inches (9 cm) wide on chairs so chair can fit under work surface
Adjustability	Up and down about 5 inches (13 cm) on chairs. Wider motion capability if armrests are on a work bench

Table B-1: Recommended Chair and Accessory Characteristics. Recommended dimensions and characteristics of chairs, footrests, and armrests are given in inches and centimeters. Few chairs will be found that possess all of the characteristics recommended; the ones that come closest are preferred.

Appendix B-Selecting a Chair 163

about the type of chair and the kind of work that is done in the seated posture, however. Figure B-1 summarizes some of the decisions that should be made before the final chair is selected. Following this process should lead one to a chair that is best suited to the job and that takes account of the usual job postures as well as the population's physical size range.

Table B-2 indicates important selection features for chairs and accessories to be used in workplaces where assembly, word processing, inspection tasks, and intermittent seated jobs are done. These tasks are described below. Each job will have its unique combination of tasks, so the chair selection process suggested in this table should be used only as a guide to how to analyze the needs.

Assembly tasks often require the worker to lean forward on the work surface in order to hold or put pressure on a part, use a tool, or attach a part to the main assembly. The operations cannot be performed while sitting back in the chair, so the backrest must be able to move forward with the worker as the work is done. Provision of workplace armrests to help steady the hands may also be desirable.

A word processing job may involve sitting back in the chair and entering text on the keyboard. There is little need to lean forward during text entry, but the word processor operator may have to go to another location to pick up the printed output. Chair height adjustability is important especially if the video display unit's keyboard is not separate from the screen. Sustained awkward head and neck postures can bring out low back pain complaints.

An inspector may remove product from the manufacturing process at some point and test it, then either return it to the line or dispose of it in a waste bin. In any case, the inspector may have to move objects around the workplace; this can include a need for frequent extended reaches, twisting of the trunk, and reaches up, down, and to the side of the primary work area. In addition, the worker may lean forward to be able to see the defects for which the inspection is being done.

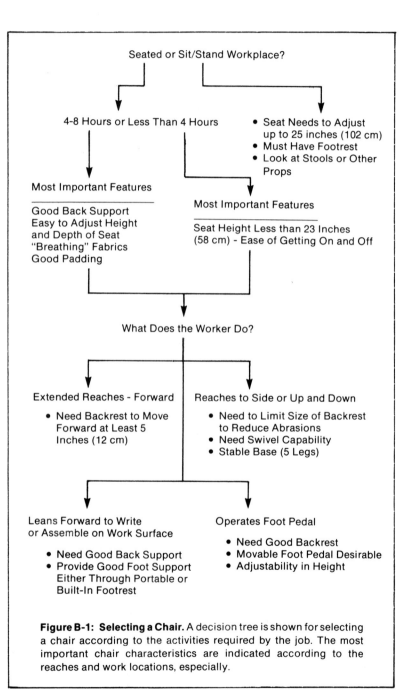

Figure B-1: Selecting a Chair. A decision tree is shown for selecting a chair according to the activities required by the job. The most important chair characteristics are indicated according to the reaches and work locations, especially.

Table B-2: Chair Selection by Job Category

Most Important Characteristics (marked by an "X")

Chair and Accessory Characteristics	Job Type			
	Assembly	Word Processing	Inspection	Seated Tasks-Intermittent
Seat Height	X	X	X	X
Seat Depth	X	X	X	X
Seat Width	X		X	
5-Legged Support	X		X	X
Backrest Size			X	
Backrest Adjustment				
Up and Down	X	X	X	X
In and Out	X		X	X
Padding	X	X	X	
Fabric Covering	X	X	X	
Footrest	X	X	X	X
Armrest	X			

Table B-2: Chair Selection by Job Category. Chair and accessory characteristics are shown in column one. Four job types are indicated across the top of the table. The most important characteristics in chair or accessory selection are marked with an "X" under each job type.

These three tasks are often done for more than 4 hours a shift and are often sustained for two hours continuously without a break. Other jobs may provide seating for people who are doing certain tasks such as paperwork, record keeping, repair work, or some testing. These intermittent seated tasks are evaluated in the last column of Table B-2.

REFERENCES

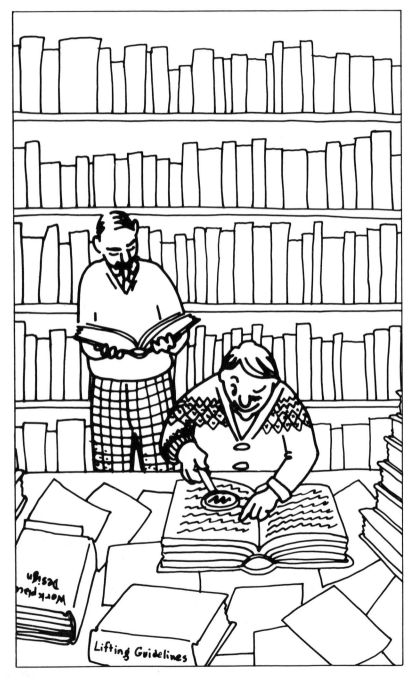

REFERENCES

Chapter 1:

Caillet, R. 1981. *Low Back Pain Syndrome. Edition 3.* Philadelphia: F.A. Davis Company, 230 pages.

Kapandji, I.A. 1974. *The Physiology of the Joints. Volume 3: The Trunk and Vertebral Column.* Translated by L.H. Honoré. New York. Churchill Livingstone, 251 pages.

Rowe, M.L. 1965. Disc surgery and chronic low back pain. *Journal of Occupational Medicine 7:* 196-202.

Rowe, M.L. 1969. Low back pain in industry. *Journal of Occupational Medicine 11:* 161-169.

Rowe, M.L. 1971. Low back disability in industry. Updated position. *Journal of Occupational Medicine 13:* 476-478.

Rowe, M.L. 1983. *Backache at Work.* Fairport, N.Y.: Perinton Press, 122 pages.

White, A.H. 1983. Back Structure, Incidence and Causative Factors of Back Injuries and Pain (Psychological, Biomechanical, and Psychophysical). Paper presented at the National Safety Council's *Back Injury Prevention and Rehabilitation Satellite Video Teleconference,* May 18, 1983. Chicago: National Safety Council, pages 7-11 of syllabus.

Chapter 2:

Chaffin, D.B. and K.S. Park. 1973. A longitudinal study of low-back pain as associated with occupational weight lifting factors. *American Industrial Hygiene Association Journal 34:* 513-525.

Kodak Human Factors. 1983. *Ergonomic Design for People at Work, Volume 1.* Belmont, Calif.: Lifetime Learning, 406 pages.

Nachemson, A. 1975. Towards a better understanding of low-back pain: A review of the mechanics of the lumbar disc. *Rheumatology and Rehabilitation 14:* 129-143.

Tichauer, E.R. 1978. *The Biomechanical Basis of Ergonomics: Anatomy Applied to the Design of Work Situations.* New York: Wiley Interscience, 99 pages.

Chapter 3:

Imrie, D. with C. Dimson. 1983. *Goodbye Backache.* New York: Arco Publishing, Inc., 159 pages.

Pfeiffer, G.J. 1983. *Self Starter. A Self Help Guide to Back Care.* Rochester, N.Y.: Xerox Corporation, 25 pages.

Rohmert, W. 1960. Zur Theorie der Erholungspausen bei dynamischer Arbeit. *Internationale Zeitschrift fur Angewandte Physiologie 18:* 191-212.

Scherrer, J. and H. Monod. 1960. Le Travail musculaire et la fatigue chez l'homme. *Journal de Physiologie (Paris) 52:* 419-501.

Chapter 4:

Brown, J.R. 1975. Factors contributing to the development of back pain in industrial workers. *American Industrial Hygiene Association Journal 36:* 26-31.

Himbury, S. 1967. *Kinetic Methods of Manual Handling in Industry.* I.L.O.: Occupational Safety and Health Series No. 10. Geneva, Switzerland: International Labour Office, 38 pages.

Chapter 5:

Chaffin, D.B. and G.B. Andersson. 1984. *Occupational Biomechanics.* New York: John Wiley & Sons, 454 pages.

Frankel, V.H. and M. Nordin. 1980. *Basic Biomechanics of the Skeletal System.* Philadelphia: Lea & Febiger, 303 pages.

Kapandji, I.A. 1974, op. cit. (Chapter 1).

Kodak Human Factors. 1983, op. cit. (Chapter 2).

NASA. 1978. *Anthropometric Source Book. Volume II: A Handbook of Anthropometric Data.* Yellow Springs, Ohio: NASA Scientific and Technical Information Office, 424 pages.

Chapter 6 and Appendix B:

Grandjean, E. 1980. *Fitting the Task to the Man: An Ergonomic Approach. 3rd Edition.* London: Taylor & Francis, Ltd., 50-62.

Grandjean, E., W. Hunting, G. Wotzka, and R. Schaerer. 1973. An ergonomic investigation of multipurpose chairs. *Human Factors 15:* 247-255.

Kodak Human Factors. 1983, op. cit. (Chapter 2).

Konz, S. 1979. *Work Design.* Columbus, Ohio: Grid Publishing Company, 592 pages.

Mandal, A.C. 1981. The seated man (Homo Sedens), the seated work position - Theory and practice. *Applied Ergonomics 12(1):* 19-26.

Roebuck, J.A. Jr., K.H.E. Kroemer, and W.G. Thomson. 1975. *Engineering Anthropometry Methods.* New York: John Wiley & Sons, 459 pages.

Chapter 7:

Astrand, P.-O. and K. Rodahl. 1977. *Textbook of Work Physiology, Second Edition.* New York: McGraw-Hill, Inc., 681 pages.

Ciriello, V. 1984. Paper presented on lifting frequency and acceptable work load at the 1984 Brouha Work Physiology Symposium in Rochester, N.Y., September, 1984.

Damon, A., H.W. Stoudt, and R.A. McFarland. 1966. *The Human Body in Equipment Design.* Cambridge, Mass.: Harvard University Press, 360 pages.

Drury, C., Editor. 1978. *Safety in Manual Materials Handling.* DHEW/NIOSH Publication No. 78-185. Cincinnati, Ohio: Department of Health, Education and Welfare/National Institute for Occupational Safety and Health, 209 pages.

Keyserling, W.M., G. Herrin, D.B. Chaffin, T.J. Armstrong, and M.L. Foss. 1980. Establishing an industrial strength testing program. *American Industrial Hygiene Association Journal 41:* 730-736.

Kroemer, K.H.E. 1970. *Horizontal Static Forces Exerted by Men Standing in Common Working Postures on Surfaces with Various Tractions.* AMRL-TR-70-114. Wright-Patterson AFB, Ohio: Aerospace Medical Research Laboratory, 36 pages.

NIOSH. 1981. *Work Practices Guide for Manual Lifting.* DHHS/NIOSH (National Institute for Occupational Safety and Health) Publication No. 81-122. Washington, D.C.: Government Printing Office, 183 pages.

Petrofsky, J.S. and A.R. Lind. 1978a. Comparison of metabolic, circulatory and ventilatory responses of man to various lifting tasks and to bicycle ergometry. *Journal of Applied Physiology (REEP) 45(1):* 60-63.

Petrofsky, J.S. and A.R. Lind. 1978b. Metabolic, cardiovascular and respiratory factors in the development of fatigue in lifting tasks. *Journal of Applied Physiology (REEP) 45(1):* 64-68.

Rohmert, W. and J. Rutenfranz. 1983. *Praktische Arbeitsphysiologie, 3rd Edition.* New York: Thieme Publishers, 440 pages.

Rowe, M.L. 1983. op. cit. (Chapter 1).

Snook, S.H. 1978. The design of manual handling tasks. *Ergonomics 21(12):* 963-985.

Snook, S.H., R.A. Campanelli, and J.W. Hart. 1978. A study of three preventive approaches to low back injury. *Journal of Occupational Medicine 20:* 478-481.

Yates, J.W. 1984. Paper on research of handling frequency and workload presented at the Brouha Work Physiology Symposium in Rochester, N.Y. in September, 1984. Paper submitted to *Ergonomics,* November 1984: Karwowski, W. and J.W. Yates. Reliability of the psychophysical approach to manual lifting of liquids by females.

Yates, J.W., E. Kamon, S.H. Rodgers, and P.C. Champney. 1980. Static lifting strength and maximum isometric voluntary contractions of back, arm, and shoulder muscles. *Ergonomics 23(1):* 37-47.

Chapter 8:

Himbury, S. 1967, op. cit. (Chapter 4).

Chapter 9:

Jacobsen, C. and L. Sperling. 1976. Classification of hand grip. A preliminary study. *Journal of Occupational Medicine 18(6):* 395-398.

Napier, S. 1956. The prehensile movements of the human hand. *Journal of Bone and Joint Surgery 38B:* 902-913.

Rigby, L.V. 1973. Why do people drop things? *Quality Progress 6(9):* 16-19.

Tichauer, E.R. 1978, op. cit. (Chapter 2).

Chapter 10:

Astrand and Rodahl. 1977, op. cit. (Chapter 7).

Lind, A.R. and J.S. Petrofsky. 1978. *Cardiovascular and Respiratory Limitations on Muscular Fatigue During Lifting Tasks.* In Drury, 1978, op. cit. (Chapter 7), pages 57-62.

Rodgers, S.H. 1978. *Metabolic Indices in Manual Materials Handling Tasks.* In Drury, 1978, op. cit. (Chapter 7), pages 52-56.

Rohmert, W. 1973a. Problems in determining rest allowances. Part 1: Use of modern methods to evaluate stress and strain in static muscle work. *Applied Ergonomics 4(2):* 91-95.

Rohmert, W. 1973b. Problems in determining rest allowances. Part 2: Determining rest allowances in different human tasks. *Applied Ergonomics 4(2):* 158-162.

Rohmert and Rutenfranz. 1983, op. cit. (Chapter 7).

Scherrer, J., H. Monod, A. Wisner, P. Andlauer, A. Baisset, S. Bouisset, H. Desoille, J.M. Faverge, A. Dubois-Poulsen, E. Grandjean, B. Metz, P. Montastruc, S. Pascaud, M. Pottier, and D. Rohr. 1967. *Physiologie du Travail (Ergonomie). Travail Physique Energetique. Volume 1.* Paris: Masson Cie., 387 pages.

Simonson, E., Compiler and Editor. 1971. *Physiology of Work Capacity and Fatigue.* Springfield, Ill.,: C.C. Thomas, 571 pages.

Chapter 11:

Salvendy, G. and M.J. Smith, Editors. 1981. *Machine Pacing and Occupational Stress.* London: Taylor & Francis Ltd., 374 pages.

INDEX

A
Action Limit (AL), NIOSH Lifting Guidelines, 98
Adjustability, Workplace Height, 118, 150
Aggravators, of Low Back Pain (LBP), 15, 19, 149, 155
Aids, to Reduce LBP, 118, 150
Anthropometric Measurements
   Seated, 71
   Standing, 70
Armrests, 88, 162
Assembly Tasks, and Chair Selection, 161

B
Back Supports, 33, 84, 113, 162
Backache at Work, by M.L. Rowe, 3, 6, 19, vii
Bending Over, 21, 66, 133
Biomechanical Stress, on Back, 21, 23, 66, 92
Body Mechanics, 66, 92

C
Capacity, Aerobic Work, 101, 135
Capacity, Muscle, 47, 92, 131
Carrying, Uneven Loading, 39, 126
Carts, for Materials Handling, 117
Chairs
   Adjustability, 81, 162
   Back Supports, 33, 84, 162
   Covering, 87, 162
   Design of, 81, 151, 162
   Lack of Foot Support, 28
   Seat Dimensions, 83, 162
   Seat Slope, 84, 162
   Selection Criteria, 151, 161
   Swivel, 31, 162
Checklist, for Workplace Survey, 155
Cost, of Low Back Pain, 10

D
Degenerative Disc Disease, 3, 149
   and Age, 8
   Natural History of, 8
Depth, of Object Handled, 126
Dimensions, of Object Handled, 124, 150
Disability, Management of in LBP, 11, 153

Disc (L5), Compressive Forces on, 19, 65, 92
Dynamic Work, Lifting, 138

E
Effort Levels, Heart Rate Elevations, 139
Exercises, for Back and Trunk Muscles, 48

F
Fatigue, Muscle, 20, 69, 131
Fitness, Back and Trunk Muscles, 48
Footrail, for Back Relief, 113
Footrests, 28, 88, 162
Foot Room, Inadequate, 37
Forces,
    Exerted, Maximum Static Pull, 95
    on L5 Disc, 19, 65, 95
    Maximum Push and Pull, 106
Frequency, Lifting, 105

G
Grip, 59, 129

H
Handholds, Design of, 129
Handling Aids, 15, 33, 41, 114, 117
Heart Rate Elevation, and Work, 139
Heavy Lifting (see Lifting)
Heavy Work, and LBP, 9
Hoists, for Materials Handling, 117
Hyperextension of Back, 22, 41, 115, 125

I
Inspection Tasks, and Chair Selection, 163
Intensity-Duration Relationship,
    Aerobic Work, 101, 138
    Muscle Work, 48, 131, 138

J
Job Design, Guidelines, 143, 146

L
Length, of Object Handled, 124
Lifting,
    Guidelines, 54, 98
    and Low Back Pain, 53, 91
    Patterns to Reduce Fatigue, 143
    Repetitive or Sustained, 43, 101, 135, 143
    Tasks, 34, 123, 135, 143, 152
    Techniques, 54, 118
    Training and LBP, 3, 14
    Two-Person, 61
Lifts, and Levelators for Handling, 118
Load,
    Oversized, 42, 124
    Size and Configuration, 124, 127
Location, of Work, 65, 92, 151
    and Backrest Use, 85
Low Back Pain,
    Aggravators, 15, 19, 149, 155
    Diagnoses, 6
    and Effort Level, 9
    Incidence, 4, 153
    Industrial Studies, 4
    and Lifting Patterns, 53, 143

Index

Management of, 11, 149
Need to Report, 9, 151

M
Manual Handling Tasks
  (see Lifting), 34, 43, 92, 118, 123, 135, 143
Muscles, for Spinal Support, 45, 65, 131

N
Nerve Root Pinch, 7, 25, 52, 131, 137
NIOSH Occasional Lift Guidelines, 98

P
Paced Work,
  and Recovery Time, 133, 143, 152
  and Slip/Trip Accidents, 159
Pallets, for Height Adjustments, 119
Patterns, of Lifting, 143
%MVC (Maximum Voluntary Contraction), 47, 131, 137
Platforms, to Adjust Working Height, 111
Postures,
  Awkward, 25, 39, 43
  Flexibility, 27, 113, 133, 146
Push and Pull Forces, 95, 106

R
Reach Extenders, 109, 152
Reaches,
  Seated, 32, 74, 150
  Standing, 23, 73, 150
Recovery Time,
  Calculations of, 137

Secondary Work,
  Breaks, 143
  from Static Work, 134
References, 169
Restrictions, Job, 44
Return to Work
  Considerations, 12

S
Seated Work,
  Constant, 33, 113
  Postures, 28
  Twisting, 30
Seating, 79, 161
Sheet Materials,
  Handling Aids, 116
Sliding,
  Instead of Lifting, 42, 60, 112
  Surfaces, Air Table, Roller Bearings, 112, 118
Slip and Trip Accidents,
  Evaluation, 159
Spasm, Muscle, 50, 132
Spine, Instability, 6, 25, 39, 131
Standing Work,
  Constant, 26, 113
  Postures, 20
Static Muscle Loading, 21, 92, 131, 137
Strength, Relative Static
  Pull, 95
  Push and Pull, 106
Supervisory Style,
  Evaluation of, 158
Survey of Workplaces, 155

T
Twisting,

    Seated, 30
    While Handling Materials,
        36, 76, 97, 112

W

Width, of Object Handled, 124
Word Processing, and
    Chair Selection, 163
Work-Recovery Cycles,
    Workload Adjustment,
        43, 60, 133, 135, 143
Workers' Compensation,
    and LBP, 3, 9, 10
Workplace Design,
    Accommodations,
        15, 65, 109
    Heights, 21, 69, 92, 111, 150
    Orientation, 30, 75, 112, 151
    Seated, 28, 80, 150, 161
    Sit/Stand, 79
    Standing, 15, 79